A Beginner's Guide to
Acupuncture

Text by Xu Mingshu

Translation by Bleanor Bouttell at BESTEASY

Cover design by Shi Hanlin

Interior design by Wang Wei

Assistant editor: Yang Wenjing

Editor: Cao Yue

ISBN: 978-1-63288-022-2

Address any comments about *A Beginner's Guide to Acupuncture* to:

SCPG

401 Broadway, Ste.1000

New York, NY 10013

USA

or

Shanghai Press and Publishing Development Co., Ltd.

Floor 5, No. 390 Fuzhou Road, Shanghai, China (200001)

Email: sppd@sppdbook.com

Printed in China by Shanghai Donnelley Printing Co., Ltd.

1   3   5   7   9   10   8   6   4   2

The material in this book is provided for informational purposes only and is not intended as medical advice. The information contained in this book should not be used to diagnose or treat any illness, disorder, disease or health problem. Always consult your physician or health care provider before beginning any treatment of any illness, disorder or injury. Use of this book, advice, and information contained in this book is at the sole choice and risk of the reader.

A Beginner's Guide to
Acupuncture

Treating Common Ailments through
Traditional Chinese Medicine

By Xu Mingshu

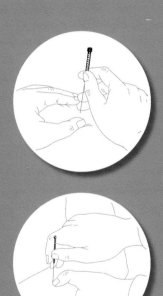

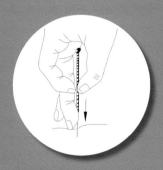

SCPG

CONTENTS

Preface

For almost three millennia, the Chinese have been practicing acupuncture and moxibustion for disease prevention and healthcare. In recent times, as cultural exchanges between East and West have flourished, acupuncture and moxibustion have become globally embraced therapeutic methods, benefiting an increasingly diverse population. Their inscription on UNESCO's Representative List of the Intangible Cultural Heritage of Humanity in 2010 is a testament to the profound cultural roots and widespread acceptance of traditional Chinese medicine.

The efficacy of acupuncture and moxibustion extends beyond addressing musculoskeletal issues, such as "neck, shoulder, back, and leg pain," to encompass various conditions in internal medicine, surgery, gynecology, pediatrics, otorhinolaryngology, ophthalmology, and stomatology. In 1996, the World Health Organization (WHO) identified 64 conditions suitable for acupuncture and moxibustion, spanning respiratory, digestive, nervous, endocrine, and musculoskeletal systems. While this book does not provide an exhaustive exploration of diseases and acupuncture points, its focus is on achieving optimal therapeutic outcomes.

Acupuncture and moxibustion, recognized for their eco-friendliness and effectiveness, merit careful study and wider promotion. However, novice acupuncturists encounter challenges such as imprecise acupuncture point location, which diminishes efficacy; incorrect needling techniques, posing potential risks; and inadequate mastery of the direction and depth of needling, particularly in critical acupuncture points.

To aid novice acupuncturists in surmounting these challenges, the book employs specific features: "quick location" with illustrations and text facilitate swift and accurate acupuncture point identification; "patterns and diagnostic features" assists in diagnosis based on primary symptoms, guiding the selection of pertinent acupuncture points for needling; "procedure of treatment" ensures precise control over needling depth, techniques, and retention time, with each step accompanied by meticulously crafted illustrations for enhanced accuracy.

It is imperative to note that due to the rigorous professional training required in acupuncture, non-medical professionals are strongly advised against attempting it independently. Those interested may explore acupuncture under the supervision of a qualified professional.

If this book proves instrumental in aiding readers' understanding of traditional Chinese medicine acupuncture, we would consider it a privilege.

CHAPTER ONE

Principles of Acupuncture Treatment

Acupuncture is a discipline that studies meridians, acupuncture points, acupuncture methods, and the laws of acupuncture prevention and treatment of diseases under the guidance of the basic theories of traditional Chinese medicine and meridian theory. It is characterized by easy operation, wide adaptability, obvious therapeutic effects, cost-effectiveness, and safety. It is not only a brilliant treasure of traditional Chinese medicine with a history spanning thousands of years, but has also been widely used in many countries around the world.

Origin of Acupuncture and Moxibustion

The formation of acupuncture has gone through a long process. When we explore its origin, there is a story circulating. Long, long ago, there was a primitive man who was hungry, so he went out to hunt. He was lucky to quickly find his prey. He charged toward and eventually killed the prey. Unfortunately, he sprained his foot during the fight. When he limped back to his dwelling dragging the prey, the pain in his ankle kept tormenting him, making it impossible for him to continue hunting. Seeing the food dwindling day by day, the primitive man began to feel anxious due to hunger, so he kept touching his ankle and praying for recovery. As the food was running out and his ankle showed no signs of improvement, the primitive man grew angry. He kept pressing and hitting the injured ankle with sharp-edged stone flakes. After a while, feeling exhausted, the starving primitive man fell asleep. When he woke up, he suddenly found that the pain in his ankle seemed to have eased. So he tried to press and hit his ankle with stone flakes again. Surprisingly, a few days later, his ankle was healed. The primitive man remembered this method and used it for treatment when injured during hunting. He found it effective and taught it to his descendants, gradually spreading it. This story might be the origin of acupuncture, but due to its ancient age, it is no longer traceable.

In the Neolithic Age, people mastered the technique of making sophisticated tools, such as needles for medical treatment, out of stone by grinding. This marks the embryonic stage of acupuncture when needling therapy was known as "*bian*-stone therapy." The stone needles used during this period are called "*bian* stone," the earliest acupuncture tools. Subsequently, bone needles, bamboo needles, and other needle tools appeared.

Moxibustion, which is often used in conjunction with acupuncture, emerged after people learned to use fire. Similar to acupuncture, moxibustion originated from the observation that certain body areas experienced relief and comfort when exposed to heat, leading to the gradual accumulation of medical knowledge. Over time, extensive practice led to refinements in materials and techniques for moxibustion, progressing from the use of assorted tree branches to the utilization of mugwort, gradually forming today's moxibustion techniques.

Acupuncture and moxibustion therapies are popular among the general public and their efficacy are well documented, so how do these therapies work?

Therapeutic Effects of Acupuncture

The acupuncture therapy is based on the philosophical theories of *yin* and *yang*, the five elements, and the theory of vital energy, and combined with the guidance of meridian theory. It stimulates acupuncture points and meridians to achieve therapeutic purposes. The therapeutic effects of acupuncture therapy are achieved through three aspects: harmonizing *yin* and *yang*, strengthening vital *qi* to eliminate pathogenic factors, and promoting the circulation of meridians.

Harmonizing *yin* and *yang*. As the cornerstone in traditional Chinese medicine, the theory of *yin* and *yang* permeates through meridians, *zang-fu* organs, etiology, pathogenesis, and syndrome differentiation and treatment. *Yin* and *yang* have opposing aspects but also interact and store each other. *Yin* and *yang* normally maintain a relatively balanced state. However, once this balance is disrupted by internal or external factors, the equilibrium of *yin* and *yang* will be relatively tilted, leading to diseases and various discomforts. Hence, the key to acupuncture treatment lies in reinforcing or reducing certain energies at the acupuncture points and meridians to regain the relative equilibrium of *yin-yang* in the body, thereby restoring normal physiological functions and treating diseases.

Strengthening vital *qi* to eliminate pathogenic factors. It refers to enhancing the body's resistance to diseases and eliminating pathogenic factors. This process involves either reinforcing the body's vital *qi* or directly expelling pathogenic factors to restore health.

Promoting the circulation of meridians. A theory of traditional Chinese medicine holds that when meridians are unobstructed, there is no pain; when there is pain, meridians are obstructed. Meridians connect the tissues and organs of the human body into an organic whole, facilitating the circulation of *qi* and blood and nourishing the whole body. Therefore, the functions of various parts of the body can be coordinated and maintained in a relative balance. When these courses are obstructed, pain occurs because *qi* and blood cannot pass through. Acupuncture and moxibustion, through various stimulation of acupuncture points on the meridians, relieve blockages and achieve the effect of treating diseases.

Acupuncture Therapy and Meridians

The concept of meridians was devised over two millennia ago. Certain scholars posit that meridians encompass the nervous system, blood vessels, lymphatic system, endocrine system, and a multi-layered, multi-functional, multi-morphological three-dimensional regulatory structure that remains incompletely comprehended. This perspective offers a more comprehensive understanding of acupuncture therapy and its mechanisms, receiving widespread acknowledgment.

The Twelve Regular Meridians

Within the human body's meridian system, there are numerous meridians and collaterals, among which the most common are the twelve regular meridians, the Governor Vessel, and the Conception Vessel along the anterior and posterior midline of the body. Below is a concise overview of the twelve regular meridians.

Naming rules of the twelve regular meridians. The twelve regular meridians are named considering the aspects of *zang-fu* organs, *yin* and *yang*, and hands and feet. *Yang* includes Shaoyang (lesser *yang*), Yangming (*yang* brightness), and Taiyang (greater *yang*); *yin* includes Shaoyin (lesser *yin*), Jueyin (reverting *yin*), and Taiyin (greater *yin*). According to traditional Chinese medicine theory, *zang* organs belong to *yin*, while *fu* organs belong to *yang*; the medial aspect is *yin*, while the lateral aspect is *yang*. The name of each meridian is based on its association with specific *zang-fu* organs and its circulation courses along the limbs. The meridians that run along the medial aspect of the limbs and belong to *zang* organs are classified as *yin* meridians, while those that run along the lateral aspect of the limbs and belong to *fu* organs are classified as *yang* meridians. For example, in the anterior aspect of the arm, the Taiyin Lung Meridian of Hand runs along the medial aspect, and the Yangming Large Intestine Meridian of Hand runs along the lateral aspect. Please refer to the table below for specific names:

Position	*Yin* Meridians	*Yang* Meridians	Circulation Courses along the Four Limbs	
	Zang Organs	*Fu* Organs	*Yin* meridians run on the medial aspect	
			Yang meridians run on the lateral aspect	
Hand	Taiyin Lung Meridian	Yangming Large Intestine Meridian	Upper limbs	Anterior aspect of the arm
	Jueyin Pericardium Meridian	Shaoyang Tripple Energizer Meridian		Medial and lateral midline of the arm
	Shaoyin Heart Meridian	Taiyang Small Intestine Meridian		Posterior aspect of the arm
Foot	Taiyin Spleen Meridian	Yangming Stomach Meridian	Lower limbs	Anterior aspect of the leg
	Jueyin Liver Meridian	Shaoyang Gallbladder Meridian		Medial and lateral midline of the leg
	Shaoyin Kidney Meridian	Taiyang Bladder Meridian		Posterior aspect of the leg

The exterior-interior relationships of the twelve meridians. The *yang* meridians and *yin* meridians in the twelve regular meridians are interconnected and complementary, forming six pairs of "exterior-interior correspondences," namely Taiyin to Yangming, Jueyin to Shaoyang, and Shaoyin to Taiyang. These pairs manifest in both hands and feet, with *yin* meridians representing the interior and *yang* meridians the superficial. Refer to the table below for specifics:

Hand	*Yin* Meridian	Taiyin Lung Meridian	Jueyin Pericardium Meridian	Shaoyin Heart Meridian	Exterior-interior correspondence
	Yang Meridian	Yangming Large Intestine Meridian	Shaoyang Tripple Energizer Meridian	Taiyang Small Intestine Meridian	
Foot	*Yang* Meridian	Yangming Stomach Meridian	Shaoyang Gallbladder Meridian	Taiyang Bladder Meridian	Exterior-interior correspondence
	Yin Meridian	Taiyin Spleen Meridian	Jueyin Liver Meridian	Shaoyin Kidney Meridian	

The circulation patterns of the twelve regular meridians. The circulation of the twelve regular meridians follow specific patterns. The three *yin* meridians of the hand all originate in the thorax and run towards the hand, intersecting with their corresponding three *yang* meridians of the hand at the fingertips. The three *yang* meridians of the hand all originate at the fingertips and run towards the head, intersecting with the three *yang* meridians of the foot on the head and face. The three *yang* meridians of foot all originate on the head and face, and run towards the foot, intersecting with their corresponding three *yin* meridians of the foot at the toes. The three *yin* meridians of foot all originate from the toes, run towards the abdomen, and then ascend to the thorax, where they intersect with the three *yin* meridians of the hand. The three *yang* meridians of the hand and foot all converge on the head and face, hence the head and face is called the "meeting point of all *yang* meridians."

Functions of Meridians

Physiological functions. ① Facilitating internal-external communication and limb connectivity. Meridians serve as conduits that integrate various bodily *zang-fu* organs and tissues into a cohesive system, ensuring harmonized bodily functions. ② Facilitating *qi* and blood circulation to nourish the entire body. The meridians can circulate *qi* and blood, distributing them throughout the body, thereby ensuring the supply of nutrients to all organs of the body and providing the necessary material foundation for the functioning of various tissues and organs. ③ Defending external pathogens and protecting the body. Nutrient *qi* flows within the meridians, while defensive *qi* circulates outside. As the meridians densely populate the skin, the defensive *qi* is densely distributed in the skin.

When the body is invaded by external pathogens, the first barriers they confront with are the skin and the hair, where the defensive *qi* plays a crucial role in defending external pathogens and protecting the body.

Pathological reflection. ① Reflecting the symptoms of the disease. The meridians, as a system that connects the internal and external aspects of the body, often manifest body's physiological dysfunctions. As certain diseases develop, obvious tenderness, nodules, streak-like reactions, or changes in the color, shape, and temperature of the corresponding skin often occur along the meridians. ② Transmitting pathogenic factors. In the state of disease, the meridians are the pathways for the transmission of pathogenic factors between the viscera and the body surface (acupuncture points). Firstly, the pathogenic factors invade the body surface (acupuncture points) and can enter the viscera through the meridians. Due to the communication between the viscera through the meridians, the pathogenic factors can also be transmitted from one viscus to another. Conversely, when the viscera are diseased, they can also be reflected in certain parts and organs of the body surface through the conduction of the meridians, showing up in the corresponding specific parts (acupuncture points), such as mouth and tongue ulcers caused by flaring up of heart fire, red and swollen eyes and ears caused by upper hyperactivity of liver fire, and deafness in both ears caused by deficiency of kidney *qi*.

Diagnostic function. Due to meridians' specific circulation areas and attachment to *zang-fu* organs, diseases in the organs and meridians can be reflected in certain areas. Therefore, the manifestations of diseases in the meridians can assist in diagnosis. In the case of headaches, meridian distribution patterns in the head can differentiate headache types. For example, frontal pain is mostly related to the Yangming meridians, pain on both sides is mostly related to the Shaoyang meridians, pain in the occipital region is mostly related to the Taiyang meridians, and pain on the top of the head is mostly related to the Jueyin meridians of foot.

In addition, obvious abnormal reactions on certain points, such as tenderness, nodules, and steak-like reactions, can help with diagnosis. Patients with appendicitis often have tenderness at the Lanwei acupoint.

Therapeutic function. The meridian theory is widely applied in the treatment of various diseases in clinical practice, especially in guiding acupuncture, moxibustion, massage, and medication therapies. In acupuncture and massage therapy, specific acupuncture points along relevant meridians are selected for treatment based on meridian or organ pathology. For example, acupuncture can be performed on relevant acupuncture points based on the location of the pain, such as using acupuncture points on the Yangming meridians for Yangming headache, and acupuncture points on the liver meridian for rib pain. In medication therapy, specific drugs are often selected to treat certain diseases based on their meridian tropism theory. For example, Chinese thorowax root (*chai hu*) is often used when there is a Shaoyang headache.

CHAPTER TWO
Precise Location of Acupuncture Points

Acupuncture points, discovered through extensive medical practice, are specific areas of the body with confirmed therapeutic effects. In ancient times, when people fell ill, they discovered, by chance, that tapping, needling, massaging, or moxibustion on painful areas could alleviate or eliminate the pain. These experiences were gradually accumulated through oral transmission. During this period, people mainly identified pain points as acupuncture points, without a precise location or specific name, which was the rudimentary stage of understanding acupuncture points.

In the long-term medical practice, people's understanding of acupuncture points has evolved. Patterns emerged, and it became apparent that certain acupuncture points had distinct locations and therapeutic applications. Descriptive accounts detailing the precise locations and associated therapeutic benefits marked its transition to a stage of localization and nomenclature.

With the advancements in understanding meridians and acupuncture points, medical practitioners of past generations have continuously summarized, analyzed, and categorized the main functions and distribution of acupuncture points, gradually categorizing acupuncture points based on their association with the fourteen meridians (the twelve regular meridians, the Conception Vessel and the Governor Vessel). As a result, acupuncture points have entered the mature stage of localization, nomenclature, and meridian tropism. Acupuncture points belonging to the fourteen meridians are called meridian points.

The number of recognized acupuncture points expanded over time. The *Inner Canon of the Yellow Emperor* (*Huangdi Neijing*) documents approximately 160 specific acupuncture point names. This number grew to 349 in the Jin dynasty (265–420), 354 in the Northern Song dynasty (960–1127), and further increased to 359 in the Ming dynasty (1368–1644), ultimately reaching 361 by the Qing dynasty (1644–1911), a count that persists to this day.

In addition to the meridian points, some acupuncture points have not been categorized within or are not suitable for classification within the fourteen meridians. These acupuncture points have specific names, clear locations, and relatively straightforward therapeutic ranges, often exhibiting special efficacy for certain diseases. They are called "extra points," such as the Sifeng acupoint for treating infantile malnutrition and the Zigong acupoint for treating gynecological disorders. While most extra points lie outside the courses of the fourteen meridians, there are exceptions, such as the Yintang and Yaoqi acupoints, which are both located on the Governor Vessel. Some extra points are combinations of meridian points, such as the "Sihua acupoints," which are composed of four acupoints including Ganshu and Danshu acupoints on both sides. Some extra points are composed of multiple points, such as the Shixuan acupoints, Bafeng acupoints, Baxie acupoints, etc.

Classification and Naming of Acupuncture Points

Acupuncture points are classified into three categories based on their fixed positions, association with the twelve regular meridians, the Conception Vessel and the Governor Vessel: fourteen meridian points, extra points, and Ashi acupoints. Please refer to the table below for details.

Classification	Name	Distribution	Meridian Tropism	Indications
Fourteen meridian points	With fixed names	Distributed on the fourteen meridian circulation courses	Belonging to the fourteen meridians	Treat diseases along the meridian circulation courses as well as diseases of the internal organs to which the meridians belong
Extra points	With fixed names	Mostly off the fourteen meridian circulation courses, but with fixed positions	Mostly not belonging to the fourteen meridians	Special therapeutic effects for certain conditions
Ashi acupoints	Without fixed names	Located based on tenderness or other reactions, often near pathological sites, but can also be distant from pathological sites, with no fixed locations; Appearing with the onset of the diseases and disappearing with the recovery of the diseases usually	Not belonging to any specific meridian	Dependent on the condition

Comprehending the names of the acupuncture points on the basis of understanding their classification facilitate familiarity with their locations, functions, and indications.

① Naming by location: that is, naming based on the anatomical location, such as the Wan'gu (Carpal Bone) acupoint besides the wrist, the Rugen (Breast Base) acupoint under the breast, and the Quanliao (Cheek Crevice) acupoint below the cheek.

② Naming by therapeutic effect: that is, naming based on the special therapeutic effect for certain conditions, such as the Jingming (Eye Bright) acupoint and Guangming (Bright Light) acupoint for treating eye diseases, the Shuifen (Water Divide) acupoint and Shuidao (Water Pathway) acupoint for treating edema, and the Qianzheng (Pull Aright) acupoint for treating facial paralysis.

③ Naming after celestial and geographical features: that is, naming based on the names of celestial bodies in the natural world, such as sun, moon, stars, and constellations, and geographical features such as mountains, streams, valleys, ponds, springs, and seas, in relation to the morphology of the acupuncture point's location or the flow of *qi* and blood, such as Riyue (Sun and Moon) acupoint, Taixi (Big Stream) acupoint, Hegu (Junction Valley) acupoint, Shuigou (Ditch) acupoint, Yongquan (Pouring Spring) acupoint, Xiaohai (Small Sea) acupoint, etc.

④ Naming after animals and plants: that is, naming based on the names of animals and plants, describing the image of the acupuncture point's location, such as Futu (Prostrate Rabbit) acupoint, Yuji (Fish Border) acupoint, Dubi (Nose of Calf) acupoint, Heding (Crane Top) acupoint, Cuanzhu (Gathering Eyebrows) acupoint, Kouheliao (Stalk Crevice) acupoint, etc.

⑤ Naming after buildings: that is, naming based on buildings to describe the morphology or functional characteristics of certain acupuncture points, such as Tianjing (Celestial Well) acupoint, Yintang (Ophryon) acupoint, Juque (Great Palace) acupoint, Dicang (Terrestrial Granary) acupoint, Liangmen (Beam Gate) acupoint, etc.

⑥ Naming according to traditional Chinese medicine theories: that is, naming based on the location or therapeutic effect of the acupuncture point, combined with the theories of *yin* and *yang*, *zang-fu* organs, meridians, *qi* and blood, etc. in traditional Chinese medicine, such as Yinlingquan (*Yin* Mound Spring) acupoint, Yanglingquan (*Yang* Mound Spring) acupoint, Xinshu (Heart *Shu*) acupoint, Sanyinjiao (Crossroad of Three *Yins*) acupoint, Baihui (Hundred Convergences) acupoint, Qihai (Sea of *Qi*) acupoint, Xuehai (Sea of Blood) acupoint, etc.

Functions of Acupuncture Points

Diagnostic function. Acupuncture points are special locations on the surface of the body where the *qi* and blood of the *zang-fu* organs and meridians are transported and accumulated. When the functions of the *zang-fu* organs and meridians in the human body are imbalanced, corresponding reflections will appear on the acupuncture points, such as tenderness, muscle swelling, concavity, cords, nodules, papules, macules, as well as changes in skin color and temperature. By observing and detecting these parts, it can assist in diagnosing diseases. For example, patients with gastrointestinal diseases often experience tenderness at acupuncture points such as Zusanli, Shangjuxu, Zhongwan, and Tianshu; patients with gynecological diseases such as dysmenorrhea often experience tenderness at acupuncture points such as Sanyinjiao, Diji, and Xuehai.

Therapeutic effects. ① Proximal therapeutic effect. This is the main therapeutic characteristic shared by all acupuncture points, which means that all acupuncture points can treat diseases of the organs and tissues in their vicinity. For example, the Jingming and Sibai acupoints around the eyes can treat eye diseases; the Zhongwan and Liangmen acupoints in the stomach area can treat stomach diseases.

② Distal therapeutic effect. This represents a fundamental principle of the primary therapeutic effects associated with the fourteen meridian points. These points, particularly those situated below the elbow and knee joints along the twelve regular meridians, exhibit the ability not only to address local ailments but also to alleviate conditions affecting distant tissues and organs along the meridians. Some acupuncture points even exert influence over systemic functions. For instance, the Hegu acupoint not only treats upper limb disorders but also addresses conditions of the neck and head, in addition to managing febrile illnesses resulting from external factors. Similarly, the Zusanli acupoint not only addresses lower limb ailments but also regulates digestive system functions and exhibits certain effects on the body's defense mechanisms and immune responses.

③ Special effects. This denotes the relative specificity and dual benign regulatory function observed in certain acupuncture points. The relative specificity of these points pertains to their specialized therapeutic effects on specific ailments, exemplified by Hegu acupoint for pain alleviation, Neiguan acupoint for nausea relief, Dazhui acupoint for fever reduction, and Zhiyin acupoint for correcting fetal positioning. Meanwhile, the dual benign regulatory function of acupuncture points signifies that stimulating a single point can yield contrasting outcomes depending on the body's state, thereby restoring equilibrium to the body's functional status. For instance, Tianshu acupoint can address both diarrhea and constipation; Neiguan acupoint can modulate heart rate by slowing it down in cases of tachycardia and accelerating it during bradycardia; Dazhui acupoint exhibits the ability to alleviate cold symptoms in wind-cold conditions and reduce fever in wind-heat ailments.

Methods for Acupuncture Points Location

The precise location of acupuncture points is critical to the clinical efficacy of acupuncture, underscoring the necessity of mastering accurate localization methods. In modern clinical practices, four primary techniques are employed to locate acupuncture points: the proportional bone measurement method, anatomical landmarks method, finger-cun measurement method, and simplified localization method.

Proportional Bone Measurement Method

The proportional bone measurement method establishes the proportional length of various body parts as the benchmark for locating acupuncture points, irrespective of gender, age, stature, or body composition. In clinical application, the proportional length of specific body regions is divided into several equal segments, each segment being termed 1 cun. For instance, the distance from the cubital crease to the wrist crease is designated as 12 cun, divided into 12 equal segments of 1 cun each. For specific measurements, please refer to the table below.

Body Part	Starting and Ending Points	Common Bone Measurement	Direction of Measurement	Explanation
Head	From middle of the front hairline to middle of the back hairline	12 cun	Vertical	If the distinction between the front and back hairlines is unclear, measure from the center of the eyebrows to the Dazhui acupoint, a distance of 18 cun.
	From the center of the eyebrows to middle of the front hairline	3 cun	Vertical	
	From Dazhui acupoint to the back hairline	3 cun	Vertical	
	Between the two hairline corners on the forehead	9 cun	Horizontal	
	Between the two mastoid processes behind the ears	9 cun	Horizontal	
Thorax and abdomen	Between the two nipples	8 cun	Horizontal	Acupuncture points in the thorax and hypochondrium are measured in vertical cun, typically calculated based on the ribs, with 1.6 cun between the upper and lower acupoints of each rib vertically. Acupuncture points in the thorax and abdomen area are measured in horizontal cun, calculated between the highest points of the two nipples into 8 cun. For females, this measurement can be adjusted by extending it up to the midpoints of the clavicles right above the two nipples.
	From the xiphisternal synchondrosis to the center of the navel	8 cun	Vertical	
	Form the center of the navel to the upper edge of the pubic symphysis	5 cun	Vertical	
Back and lumbar	From below the Dazhui acupoint to the coccyx	21 vertebras	Vertical	The vertical measurements of the back are determined by the vertebrae of the spine, where the lower angle of the scapula corresponds to the spinous process of the 7th (thoracic) vertebra spinous process, and the iliac crest aligns with the spinous process of the 16th vertebra (spinous process of the 4th lumbar vertebra).
	Medial edge of the scapula	6 cun	Horizontal	

Body Part	Starting and Ending Points	Common Bone Measurement	Direction of Measurement	Explanation
Upper limbs	From the anterior axillary fold to cubital crease	9 cun	Vertical	Used for bone measurement of the three *yin* meridians of hand and three *yang* meridians of hand.
	From the cubital crease to the wrist crease	12 cun	Vertical	
Lower limbs	From the upper edge of the pubic bone to the upper edge of the medial condyle of the femur	18 cun	Vertical	Used for bone measurement of the three *yin* meridians of foot; the upper edge of the medial condyle of the femur is at the same level as the bottom of the patella.
	From below the condylus medialis tibiae to prominence of the medial malleolus	13 cun	Vertical	
	From the greater trochanter of the femur to the middle of the knee	19 cun	Vertical	Used for bone measurement of the three *yang* meridians of foot; the anterior aspect of middle of the knee corresponds to the Dubi acupoint, and the posterior aspect corresponds to the Weizhong acupoint; from the gluteal sulcus to the middle of the knee, it measures 14 cun.
	From the middle of the knee to the prominence of the lateral malleolus	16 cun	Vertical	

Anatomical Landmarks Method

This method is divided into fixed landmarks and active landmarks.

Fixed landmarks. Fixed landmarks are those unaffected by human movement and remain stationary. These include facial features, hair, nails, nipples, umbilicus, and various bone protrusions and depressions. For instance, the Suliao acupoint is located at the tip of the nose, the Yintang acupoint is found between the eyebrows, and the Danzhong acupoint is situated between the nipples. In addition, anatomical landmarks, such as the 3rd thoracic spinous process aligned with the scapular spine, the 7th thoracic spinous process aligned with the lower angle of the scapula, and the 4th lumbar spinous process aligned with the iliac crest, can be used to locate acupuncture points on the lower back.

Active landmarks. Active landmarks require specific movements to identify. For example, to locate the Ermen, Tinggong and Tinghui acupoints, open the mouth and press the depression in front of the tragus; to locate the Yangxi acupoint, raise the thumb and press the depression between the extensor digitorum longus tendon and the extensor digitorum brevis of the thumb; to locate the Houxi acupoint, make a fist and find the point at the end of the transverse line of the palm.

Finger-cun Measurement Method

This is a technique used to measure and locate acupuncture points using the patient's fingers as a standard.

① Thumb-cun measurement: The width of the patient's thumb joint is used as 1 cun. This method is suitable for measuring and locating acupuncture points on the limbs vertically.

② Middle finger-cun measurement: Take the distance between the two transverse lines at the inner ends of the middle joint of the patient's middle finger when flexed as 1 cun. This method can be used to locate acupuncture points on the limbs vertically and on the back horizontally.

③ Four finger-cun measurement: With the index finger, middle finger, ring finger, and small finger of the patient stretched straight and closed, measure at the level of the large knuckle (the second joint) of the middle finger. The width of the four fingers is 3 cun. This method can be used to locate acupuncture points on the limbs vertically and transverse points on the back horizontally.

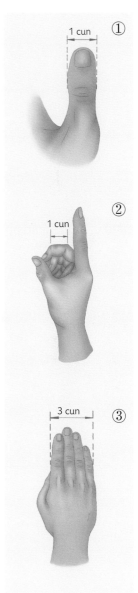

Simplified Localization Method

In clinical practice, a commonly used simple and practical method for locating acupuncture points involves techniques such as: taking the midpoint of the line connecting the two ear tips as the Baihui acupoint; intersecting the web between the thumb and index finger of both hands to locate the Lieque acupoint; finding the Fengshi acupoint where the tip of the middle finger touches the thigh when hanging down; and dropping the shoulder and bending the elbow to identify the Zhangmen acupoint. These methods are summarized based on long-term clinical practice.

CHAPTER THREE
Acupuncture and Moxibustion Techniques

Acupuncture and moxibustion are two independent and distinctive external therapeutic modalities in traditional Chinese medicine. Acupuncture involves mechanical stimulation, while moxibustion employs warm stimulation. Mastery of techniques is crucial for achieving optimal therapeutic effects through these methods. This chapter delves into the nuances of acupuncture and moxibustion techniques.

Acupuncture Techniques

There are various techniques for needling, and choosing and mastering the right technique is the key.

Acupuncture Practice

For beginners, practicing needling is indispensable and primarily focuses on finger strength and technique. Insufficient finger strength may result in slow penetration of the needle tip, causing pain to the patient. Additionally, inadequate proficiency in needling technique may lead to needle retention during twirling manipulation, resulting in unexpected outcomes. Here are several common methods for practicing needling techniques:

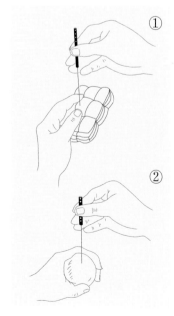

① Practicing needling techniques on paper pads: Fold soft paper into an 8 cm × 5 cm (length × width) block. The thickness of the paper block can be adjusted based on individual proficiency levels, ranging from 2 to 3 cm for beginners to 3 to 5 cm for those with stronger finger strength. Tie the paper block with cotton thread into a "#" shape to create a paper pad and compact it. Various needle insertion techniques can be repeatedly practiced on the paper pad.

② Practicing needling techniques on cotton balls: Wrap a lump of cotton wool in cloth and tie it tightly with a rubber band to make a cotton ball 6 to 7 cm in diameter. The needle practice method is the same as that on the paper pad. The softness of the cotton ball allows for practicing various basic needling techniques such as lifting and thrusting method and twirling method.

③ Practicing needling techniques on a skin model: Skin models, available for purchase, usually consist of a low-resistance zone and a high-resistance zone catering to different needs. This method is similar to practicing on paper pads.

Preparation before Needling

Selection of needles: In clinical practice, appropriate needles of suitable length and thickness should be selected based on the patient's gender, age, body size, constitution, condition, affected area, and selected acupuncture points. For example, for males who are muscular, overweight with deep disease location, slightly thicker and longer filiform needles may be preferred. Conversely, for females who are slender, delicate with superficial disease location, shorter and thinner needles are recommended. Thin-skinned areas and shallow acupuncture points should be treated with short and fine needles, while thick-skinned areas require longer and thicker needles. Additionally, after inserting the needle to the appropriate depth into the acupuncture point, the needle body should still protrude slightly from the skin.

Selection of positions: Before acupuncture, a relatively comfortable position that the patient can tolerate for a longer period of time should be selected based on the chosen acupuncture points and the patient's actual condition. This not only facilitates the procedure, but also allows for appropriate needle retention and prevents various abnormal situations caused by the patient changing positions during the acupuncture process. Commonly used acupuncture positions in clinical practice include reclining with back support, prone sitting, supine lying, lateral lying, and prone lying. For patients with initial diagnosis, mental tension, or old age, weakness, and serious illness, it is advisable to adopt a lying position.

Disinfection: With the prevalent use of disposable sterilized acupuncture needles in modern clinical settings, the disinfection of needles is relatively simple. Before use, it is essential to verify the needles' expiration date. If they are within the validity period, take out the disposable sterilized acupuncture needles from the sealed package and use them. However, it should be noted that once the sealed packaging is opened, the needles should be utilized promptly. In the event of unused needles, they can be soaked in 75% alcohol for 30 minutes for disinfection before subsequent use. Acupuncture points can be disinfected by wiping with a 75% alcohol-soaked cotton ball, starting from the center and wiping in a circular motion; or first wiping with 2.5% iodine tincture, and then wiping off the iodine tincture with a 75% alcohol-soaked cotton ball. Regarding the disinfection of a practitioner's fingers, it is recommended to first wash them with soapy water and then wipe them down with a 75% alcohol-soaked cotton ball.

Needle Holding Postures

Most clinical practitioners hold the needle with their right hand while using their left hand to assist in needle insertion. The needle holding postures involve different combination of fingers, such as thumb and index finger, thumb and middle finger, and thumb, index finger and middle finger together. One can also hold the needle body.

① Using thumb and index finger: Hold the needle handle with the right thumb and index finger to perform needling.

② Using thumb and middle finger: Hold the needle handle with the right thumb and middle finger to perform needling.

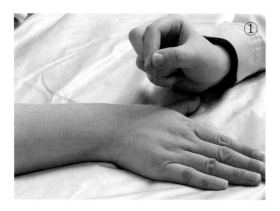
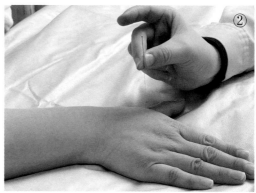

③ Using thumb, index, and middle fingers together: Hold the needle handle with the distal phalanx of the right thumb, index finger, and middle finger, with the thumb inside and the index and middle fingers outside, to perform needling.

④ Holding the needle body: Hold a sterilized dry cotton ball with the right thumb and index finger, wrap it around the end of the needle close to the needle tip, to perform needling.

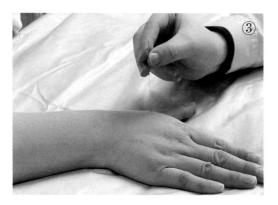
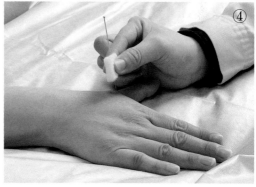

Needle Inserting Methods

Needle-inserting method with a single hand. Hold the lower part of the needle handle with the thumb and index finger of the right hand. The pulp of the middle finger, positioned against the lower portion of the needle body, extends slightly beyond or aligns evenly with the needle tip. With precision alignment to the acupuncture point, the tip of the middle finger firmly presses against the skin, while the thumb and index finger apply downward pressure with the middle finger bended to

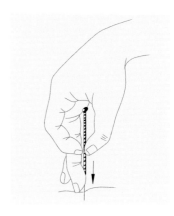

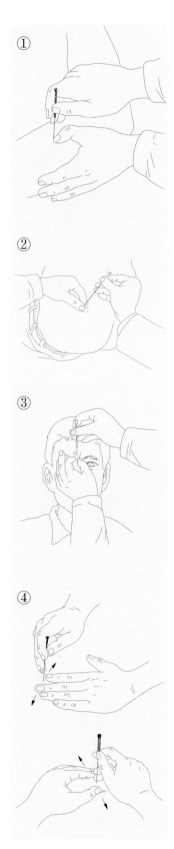

insert the needle swiftly, ensuring that the needle remains straight throughout insertion.

Needle-inserting method with both hands.

① Fingernail-pressure needle inserting method: With the thumb or index finger of the left hand, apply pressure adjacent to the acupuncture point to stabilize it. Hold the needle handle with the pulp of the thumb, index finger, and middle finger of the right hand, ensuring the needle is perpendicular to the skin surface, pressing it closely against the nail surface of the left hand and swiftly insert it. This technique is suitable for short needle insertions.

② Insertion of the needle by holding needle tip with thumb and index finger: Grasp the lower part of the needle with the thumb and index finger of the left hand, wrapped in a sterilized dry cotton ball (leaving 0.3 to 0.5 cm of the needle tip exposed). With the pulp of the thumb, index finger, and middle finger of the right hand, hold the needle handle, keeping the needle perpendicular to the skin surface. Fix the needle tip on the surface of the acupuncture point, twirl the needle handle with the right hand, press down with the left hand, and coordinate both hands to swiftly insert the needle into the subcutaneous tissue. This technique is suitable for long needle insertions.

③ Skin-pinching needle inserting method: Gently pinch the skin near the acupuncture point with the thumb and index finger of the left hand, ensuring appropriate pressure; hold the needle handle with the pulp of the thumb, index finger, and middle finger of the right hand, and quickly insert the needle into the acupuncture point. This technique is suitable for shallow acupuncture points in thin-skinned areas. It is often combined with horizontal insertion. (see page 29).

④ Skin-stretching needle inserting method: Use the thumb and index finger, or index and middle finger of the left hand to gently stretch the skin at the acupuncture point, making it taut. The distance between the two fingers should be appropriate. Hold the needle handle with the thumb, index finger, and middle finger of the right hand, and quickly insert it into the acupuncture point between the two fingers of the left hand. This method is suitable for needle insertion at acupuncture points in loose-skinned areas.

Direction, Angle, and Depth of Needling

Mastering the correct direction, angle, and depth during needling is pivotal for its efficacy and prevents any procedural anomalies. Different needling sensations and therapeutic effects can arise from varying angles, directions, and depths of needle insertion at the same acupuncture point.

Direction of needling. This refers to a certain direction or position targeted by the needle tip during insertion. Generally, the direction of the needle tip follows the course of the twelve regular meridians (refer to page 14), with a direction consistent with the meridian circulation courses for reinforcement and the opposite for reduction. In addition, some acupuncture points have special locations, and special attention should be paid to the direction when needling. For example, when needling the Fengchi acupoint, the needle tip should be slowly inserted towards the tip of the nose; when targeting the Tiantu acupoint, initially insert the needle 0.2 cun deep, and upon surpassing the inner edge of the manubrium sterni, proceed to insert it downwards along the medial edge of the manubrium sterni and the anterior edge of the trachea for 0.5 to 1 cun. Furthermore, adjusting the needle tip's direction towards the affected area during needling is crucial for achieving the desired effect, i.e., "allowing *qi* to reach the affected area."

Angle of needling. This refers to the angle formed between the needle body and the skin surface during insertion, generally categorized into perpendicular insertion, oblique insertion and horizontal insertion. Specifically as follows:

Designation	Perpendicular insertion	Oblique insertion	Horizontal insertion
Angle of Needle Insertion	The needle is inserted perpendicular to the skin surface at a 90° angle.	The needle is inserted at an angle of approximately 45° to the skin surface.	The needle is inserted at an angle of approximately 15° to the skin surface.
Applicable Body Parts	Applicable to most acupuncture points.	Applicable to acupuncture points in areas with shallow muscles or important organs inside, or acupuncture points that are not suitable for perpendicular or deep needling.	Applicable to acupuncture points in thin-skinned areas, such as acupuncture points on the head.

Depth of needling. This refers to the depth of needling into the human body, depending on the patient's age, constitution, condition, and body part. Specifically as follows:

Designation	Age	Constitution	Condition	Body Part
Deep insertion	Middle-aged and young individuals	Those with strong bodies or overweight	Interior syndrome, deficiency syndrome, cold syndrome, chronic illness	Limbs, buttocks, abdomen, and muscular areas
Shallow insertion	Elderly and weak individuals, as well as children	Those with weak bodies	Exterior syndrome, excess syndrome, heat syndrome, new diseases	Head, face, thorax and back, and areas with thin skin and little flesh

The angle and depth of needling are closely related. Generally, perpendicular insertion is used for deep needling, and oblique or horizontal insertion is used for shallow needling. For acupuncture points such as Tiantu, Yamen, Fengchi, Fengfu, and eye area, as well as acupuncture points in the thorax, back, and important organs such as the heart, liver, and lungs, special attention should be paid to mastering the angle and depth of needling.

Acupuncture Techniques

This refers to the various methods employed by practitioners on acupuncture points from the insertion of the needle to its withdrawal, aiming to facilitate the patient's *qi* flow or enhance needling sensation.

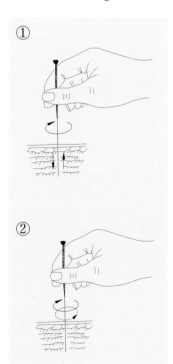

①

②

Basic methods. ① Lifting and thrusting method. This method involves inserting the needle into the acupuncture point to a certain depth and then manipulating it up and down, i.e., inserting it to a deeper layer (thrusting), and withdrawing it to a shallow layer (lifting). The amplitude, frequency, and duration of the lifting and thrusting should be determined according to the patient's constitution, condition, and the location of the acupuncture point.

② Twirling method. This method involves inserting the needle into the acupuncture point to a certain depth, holding the needle handle with the thumb and middle finger or index finger of the right hand, and twirling it back and forth. The angle, frequency, and duration of twirling are consistent with the lifting and thrusting method.

The lifting and thrusting method and the twirling method can be utilized independently or combined, offering flexibility to adapt to various situations.

Auxiliary methods. ① Mild pressing along meridian course method. Use the hand to press or tap along the meridian or around the acupuncture point to promote blood circulation and the flow of *qi* in the meridian.

Specific procedure: Insert the needle into the acupuncture point to a certain depth. Utilize the pulp of the thumb or, by bringing the 2nd to 4th fingers together, employ the pulp of the 3rd finger. Press or tap along the meridian course or the areas up, down, left, and right of the acupuncture point. Repeat several times. This method is frequently applied for patients experiencing delayed or absent *qi* response after needle insertion. It can also enhance the needling sensation.

② Handle-flicking method. This refers to the method of gently tapping the needle handle with the fingers after insertion to create a subtle vibration in the needle body, aiming to promote the flow of *qi* in the meridian.

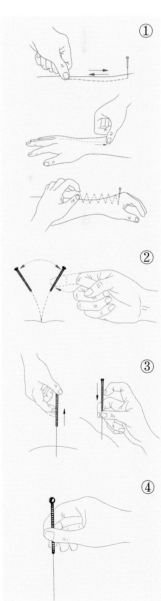

Specific procedure: Insert the needle into the acupuncture point to a certain depth, form a ring shape with the thumb and index finger, and lightly press the index fingernail against the pulp of the thumb. Align the index fingernail with the needle handle or tip, and gently flick it to induce a slight vibration in the needle body. Alternatively, use the thumb and other fingers to tap several times. This method is frequently applied for patients experiencing delayed or absent *qi* response after needle insertion or for those unable to lift, thrust or twirl the needle due to tense muscles or other conditions. It can also enhance the needling sensation.

③ Handle-scraping method. This refers to the method of stimulating the meridian *qi* and assisting the flow of *qi* by scraping the needle handle after the needle is inserted.

Specific procedure: Insert the needle into the acupuncture point to a certain depth, gently press the needle tail with the pulp of the thumb or index finger, and scrape the needle handle frequently with the fingernail of the index finger, thumb, or middle finger. The needle handle can be scraped from the base to the top or vice versa, inducing a mild vibration in the needle body. Repeat the scraping several times. This technique is suitable for patients with a weak constitution, excessive mental tension, fatigue, heightened sensitivity, or those visiting for the first time. It can also enhance the needling sensation.

④ Handle-twisting method. This refers to the method of twirling the needle in one direction with the fingers while simultaneously employing the lifting and thrusting method.

Specific procedure: Insert the needle into the acupuncture point to a certain depth, hold the needle handle with the thumb, index finger, and middle finger of the right hand, and twirl it in one direction like rubbing a thread, for 2 to 3 rounds or 3 to 5 rounds each time. Then, insert the needle into a deeper layer or withdraw it to a shallow layer, and the single-direction twirling motion is repeated to prevent the needle from entangling the muscle fibers. This method promotes the flow of *qi* in the meridian, reinforcing deficiency and reducing excess.

⑤ Handle-waggling method. After the needle is inserted, hold the needle handle and waggle it.

Specific procedure: Perpendicular needle waggling: Insert the needle perpendicularly into the acupuncture point to a certain depth, hold the needle handle, waggle it in a circular motion, or waggle it back and forth or left and right. Repeat several times.

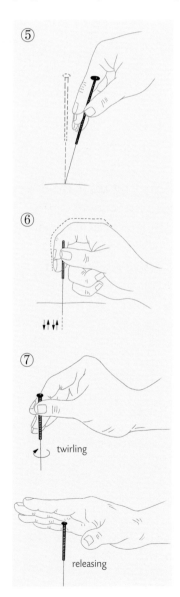

Reclining needle waggling: Insert the needle obliquely or horizontally into the acupuncture point to a certain depth, hold the needle handle, and waggle it left and right. Repeat several times. This method promotes the flow of *qi* in the meridian, enhances the needling sensation, and expels pathogenic factors.

⑥ Trembling method. This refers to the method of inserting the needle and using the hand to hold the needle handle to perform small-amplitude, high-frequency lifting, thrusting, and twirling, inducing slight trembling of the needle body.

Specific procedure: Insert the needle into the acupuncture point to a certain depth, hold the needle handle with the thumb and index finger or thumb, index finger, and middle finger of the right hand, and perform small-amplitude, high-frequency lifting, thrusting, and twirling, resembling hand tremors. Repeat several times. This method promotes the flow of *qi* in the meridian, enhances needling sensation, and strengthens the body to expel pathogenic factors.

⑦ Flying method. This refers to the method of inserting the needle and then twirling the needle handle several times before suddenly releasing the fingers to create a trembling effect.

Specific procedure: Insert the needle into the acupuncture point to a certain depth, hold the needle handle with the thumb and index finger or thumb, index finger, and middle finger, and twirl and release the needle.

While twirling, curl the index and middle finger inward to rotate the needle clockwise; while releasing, extend the index and middle finger outward and rub the needle handle to rotate the needle counterclockwise. Repeat several times. Then quickly release the fingers to make the needle tremble like a bird spreading its wings. Repeat several times. This method promotes the flow of *qi* in the meridian and enhances the needling sensation. It is suitable for patients who fear needles and experience muscle spasms and pain.

Qi Sensation from Needling

Qi sensation from needling, also known as needling sensation, refers to the meridian *qi* response generated at the site of needle insertion after reaching a certain depth or applying techniques such as lifting and thrusting or twirling the needle. With *qi* sensation, the practitioner may perceive a sense of smoothness or heaviness under the needle; while the patient may experience sensations such as soreness, numbness, swelling, and heaviness at the needle insertion site. In addition, some patients may experience sensations of conduction and diffusion in specific directions and areas, or exhibit meridian-related muscle tremors, involuntary limb movements, or skin reactions such as rashes or red and white lines. Sensations of heat, cold, itching, electric shock, airflow, water waves, jumping, ant crawling, convulsions, and pain are all indicative of *qi* sensation from needling. Conversely, without *qi* sensation, the practitioner will feel emptiness under the needle, and the patient will not experience any sensations such as soreness, numbness, swelling, heaviness, or others.

The presence or absence of *qi* sensation from needling is directly related to the therapeutic effect of acupuncture. In general, a swift *qi* sensation corresponds to better therapeutic outcomes, whereas a slow *qi* sensation results in poorer effects. In addition, the presence or absence of *qi* sensation from needling can also predict the prognosis of the disease. Patients who fail to acquire *qi* sensation even after repeated application of needling techniques often suffer from depleted vital *qi*, indicating an extremely poor prognosis. However, if initial treatments fail to elicit *qi* sensation or result in slow *qi* sensation, but subsequent correct application of needling techniques leads to swift *qi* sensation, it signifies the restoration of vital *qi* in the patient and a favorable prognosis.

Acupuncture Reinforcement and Reduction

① Reinforcing method. This refers to the method that invigorates the vital *qi* of the human body and boosts weakened functions.

② Reducing method. This refers to the method that promotes the elimination of pathogenic factors and dissipates excessive functions to normalcy.

Acupuncture reinforcement and reduction involve stimulating meridian *qi* through acupuncture points by utilizing appropriate techniques to benefit the vital *qi*, eliminate pathogenic factors, and regulate *zang-fu* organs and meridian functions, thereby promoting the balance of *yin* and *yang* and restoring health. Please refer to the table on the next page for common acupuncture reinforcement and reduction methods.

Reinforcing and Reducing Methods	Specific Procedure	
	Reinforcing Method	Reducing Method
Reinforcing-reducing method by twirling	With *qi* sensation from needling, twirl the needle by applying force with the thumb forward and the index finger backward. Maintain a small twirling angle, slow frequency, and gentle force. Repeat the twirling briefly.	With *qi* sensation from needling, twirl the needle by applying force with the thumb backward and the index finger forward. Maintain a large twirling angle, fast frequency, and heavy force. Repeat the twirling for a prolonged duration.
Reinforcing-reducing method by lifting-thrusting	With *qi* sensation from needling, first insert the needle shallowly then deeply, applying heavy thrusting and light lifting. Maintain a small amplitude of lifting-thrusting, slow frequency, and short duration. Swiftly and firmly thrust the needle, and slowly and gently lift it.	With *qi* sensation from needling, first insert the needle deeply then shallowly, applying light thrusting and heavy lifting. Maintain a large amplitude of lifting-thrusting, fast frequency, and prolonged duration. Slowly and gently thrust the needle, and swiftly and firmly lift it.
Slow-rapid reinforcing-reducing method	During needle insertion, slowly push the needle inward to a certain depth, refrain from any needle manipulation during needle retention, and swiftly withdraw the needle to the subcutaneous tissue.	Quickly insert the needle to the required depth during needle insertion, perform needle manipulation during needle retention, and slowly withdraw the needle.
Directional reinforcing-reducing method	Insert the needle tip along the direction of the meridian course.	Insert the needle tip against the direction of the meridian course.
Respirational reinforcing-reducing method	Insert the needle when the patient exhales and withdraw it when the patient inhales.	Insert the needle when the patient inhales and withdraw it when the patient exhales.
Open-closed reinforcing-reducing method	Quickly close the needle hole after withdrawing the needle.	Upon needle withdrawal, widen the needle hole with a gentle shake, refraining from applying any pressure to close it.
Even reinforcing-reducing method	With the arrival of *qi*, apply a uniform and slow lifting, thrusting, and twirling technique, ensuring consistent amplitude and angle, moderate frequency, smooth rhythm, and appropriate needling sensation.	

Needle retention method. The needle retention method refers to the practice of retaining the needle in the acupuncture point for a specific duration after achieving the desired *qi* sensation to enhance the needling sensation and prolong the effect of acupuncture.

Whether to retain the needle and the duration of needle retention should be determined based on the patient's constitution, condition, and the location of the acupuncture point. For general conditions, once the desired *qi* sensation is achieved and appropriate reinforcing or reducing methods are applied, the needle can be withdrawn, or it can be retained for 10 to 30 minutes. However, for chronic, stubborn, painful, and spasmodic conditions, the retention time can be increased accordingly. Note that needle retention should be avoided for extended periods in elderly, pediatric, and frail patients, while it may be extended for younger and stronger patients. Acupuncture points in the posterior head, eye area, throat, and thorax and back should not be retained for a long time. In addition, for patients who do not achieve the desired *qi* sensation with various acupuncture techniques, needle retention can be utilized to await the arrival of *qi*.

There are two types of needle retention: dynamic and static. Dynamic needle retention involves leaving the needle in place for a certain period after achieving *qi* sensation, during which intermittent needling techniques are applied to enhance the needling sensation and the therapeutic effects of reinforcing deficiency or reducing excess. It can be further categorized into short-term and long-term methods based on the duration of retention. Short-term dynamic needle retention typically lasts for 10 to 30 minutes with intermittent needling 1 to 3 times, while long-term dynamic needle retention may last for several hours while needling once every 10 to 30 minutes. For patients who fail to achieve *qi* sensation from needling, dynamic needle retention can be used to promote *qi* flow to the needle.

However, it is important to note that dynamic needle retention should be avoided for uncooperative children, needle-phobic patients, first-time acupuncture recipients, and patients with extremely weak constitutions. In addition, dynamic needle retention should not be used on acupuncture points in the eye area, throat area, and thorax area. Some diseases, such as frequent urination, urgent urination, and coughing and wheezing, should also not be treated with dynamic needle retention.

Static needle retention refers to the needle being inserted into the body and naturally staying in place for a period of time without applying any needling techniques. Static needle retention is suitable for patients with poor tolerance to needling sensation and those with a weaker constitution.

Needle withdrawal method. This refers to the practice of withdrawing the needle from the body after achieving *qi* sensation or been retained for a specified duration to meet treatment requirements. During needle withdrawal, the skin around the needle hole is gently pressed with a dry sterilized cotton ball using the thumb and index finger of the left hand. With the right hand, the needle is carefully twirled and lifted to the subcutaneous tissue, followed by a swift removal. Subsequently, a dry sterilized cotton ball is applied to the hole for a brief moment to prevent bleeding. Finally, it is imperative to conduct a thorough check to ensure no needles are inadvertently left behind.

Handling of Accidents

While acupuncture therapy is generally safe, improper operation may lead to abnormal situations. It is essential to properly address any abnormal occurrences.

⋆ Fainting

Causes: Fainting commonly occurs in patients undergoing acupuncture for the first time. It is often attributed to mental tension, weak constitution, hunger, excessive fatigue, profuse sweating, diarrhea, excessive bleeding, improper positioning, or excessive needle manipulation, resulting in temporary cerebral ischemia during acupuncture or the needling process.

Symptoms: Patients may suddenly experience mental fatigue, dizziness, pallor, palpitations, shortness of breath, nausea, cold sweats, cold extremities, decreased blood pressure, and a deep, thready pulse. Severe cases may involve loss of consciousness, collapse, cyanosis of the lips and nails, urinary or fecal incontinence, and an almost imperceptible pulse.

Treatment: Immediately cease acupuncture, remove all needles, and position the patient in a supine position with the head slightly lowered while loosening tight clothing and ensuring warmth. Mild cases may be managed with rest and oral intake of warm water or sugar water. For severe cases, in addition to the aforementioned measures, acupressure or needling at Renzhong, Suliao, Neiguan, Hegu, Taichong, Yongquan, and Zusanli acupoints, or moxibustion at Baihui, Qihai and Guanyuan acupoints can be performed. If necessary, other emergency interventions should be considered.

Prevention: Patients receiving acupuncture for the first time or those experiencing mental tension should be thoroughly informed about the procedure to alleviate concerns. Comfortable and enduring positioning (preferably a lying position), limited acupuncture points, and gentle manipulation are recommended. Acupuncture should be avoided for individuals experiencing severe hunger or fatigue. Continuous monitoring of the patient's condition and early recognition of pre-fainting symptoms are essential for prompt intervention.

⋆ Sticking of Needle

Causes: The patient may experience mental tension or pain, resulting in strong local muscle contraction after needle insertion. Additionally, the needle may become stuck if inserted into a tendon, twirled at an excessive angle, or continuously twirled in one direction, causing entanglement of muscle fibers around the needle. Prolonged needle retention can also lead to sticking of the needle.

Symptoms: After needle insertion, it becomes challenging to manipulate techniques such as lifting and thrusting, twirling the needle, and withdrawing the needle becomes difficult.

Treatment: Advise the patient to relax and avoid tension in the local muscles. If the needle is stuck due to excessive twirling, gently twirl the needle back in the opposite direction. If the patient is mentally tense or experiences muscle spasms, retain the needle in place for a period before attempting to withdraw it. Alternatively, massage the surrounding area or insert another needle nearby to distract the patient's attention before withdrawing the stuck needle.

Prevention: Make sure that patients with mental tension are well informed about the procedure to alleviate concerns. When inserting the needle, avoid tendons, and ensure that the twirling angle is not too large, refraining from continuous twirling in one direction.

★ Bending of Needle

Causes: The practitioner's needling technique may be unskilled, resulting in excessive force or encountering hard tissues during insertion. Additionally, a patient's change in position during needle retention or external pressure and collision on the needle handle can cause bending. Failure to address stuck needles promptly and correctly can also lead to bending.

Symptoms: The needle body is bent, and the needle handle changes the direction and angle of insertion, making it challenging to use techniques such as lifting and thrusting, twirling, leading to difficult needle withdrawal, and causing pain to the patient.

Treatment: If the bending is slight, making lifting and thrusting, twirling procedures impossible, slowly withdraw the needle; if the bending angle is too large, the needle should be withdrawn along the bending direction; if it is caused by a change in the patient's position, the patient should be instructed to return to the original position to relax the local muscles before withdrawing the needle, and avoid forcefully pulling out the needle.

Prevention: Practitioners should use proficient techniques with gentle finger pressure, ensure patient comfort during needle insertion, avoid random changes in position during needle retention, and prevent external collision and pressure on the needle insertion site and handle. Prompt and correct handling of stuck needles is essential to prevent bending.

★ Fracture of Needle

A fracture of needle refers to a situation where the needle body breaks inside the patient's body. Due to the advancement in needle manufacturing technology and the widespread use of disposable sterilized acupuncture needles, needle fracture incidents have become extremely rare in clinical practice.

Causes: Poor needle quality, erosion, or damage to the needle body or root; inserting the entire needle body during needling; strong twirling, lifting and thrusting forces causing intense muscle contraction in the patient; patient changing position while the needle is retained; failure to promptly and correctly handle stuck or bent needles.

Symptoms: The needle body breaks, leaving a fragment inside the patient's body.

Treatment: Calm the patient and advise against moving to prevent the broken end from penetrating deeper into the muscle. If the fragment is outside the body, remove it with fingers or tweezers; if it is level with the skin, squeeze the needle holes on both sides to expose the fragment for removal with tweezers; if the needle body is completely embedded in the muscle, locate it under X-ray and surgically remove it.

Prevention: Purchase needles from reputable sources and carefully inspect them before use. Avoid inserting the entire needle body during needling; avoid excessive force during needling; instruct patients not to change positions randomly during needling or needle retention; withdraw the needle immediately if it bends during needling; handle stuck or bent needles promptly and correctly without forceful removal.

★ Hematoma

Cause: The needle tip is bent with a hook, causing damage to the skin or puncturing blood vessels when needling.

Symptoms: Swelling, pain, or bleeding at the acupuncture site after needle withdrawal, followed by local purplish-blue skin.

Treatment: Minor subcutaneous bleeding or small bruising at the needle hole are caused by damage to small blood vessels. They can usually resolve on their own and do not require treatment. For severe swelling, pain, or large bruising affecting function, apply a cold compress to stop bleeding first, then a hot compress or local massage after 48 hours to promote blood stasis dissipation.

Prevention: Thoroughly inspect needles, get familiarized with anatomical sites, avoid puncturing blood vessels, and press the needle hole with a dry disinfectant cotton ball when withdrawing the needle.

Contraindications for Acupuncture

① Patients who are excessively hungry, excessively fatigued, or highly mentally stressed should not undergo immediate acupuncture. For patients with weak constitution and deficiency of *qi* and blood, acupuncture techniques should not be strong, and lying position should be adopted whenever possible.

② Pregnant women's abdomen, lumbosacral region, and some acupuncture points that can cause uterine contractions such as Hegu, Sanyinjiao, Kunlun, and Zhiyin acupoints should not be needled. During menstruation, acupuncture should generally be avoided unless specifically for menstrual regulation.

③ When the fontanelle of an infant is not closed, the acupuncture points on the top of the head should not be needled. In addition, if the child cannot cooperate, it is also not suitable for needle retention.

④ Patients with spontaneous bleeding or persistent bleeding after injury should not be needled.

⑤ Needle insertion is not suitable for areas with skin infections, ulcers, scars, or tumors.

⑥ Avoid hurting important organs.

a. When needling acupuncture points in the eye area, precise angles and depths should be maintained. Avoid excessive lifting and thrusting, twirling, or retaining the needle for a long period of time to prevent injury to the eyeball and bleeding.

b. For the acupuncture points on both sides of the 11th thoracic vertebra on the back, the 8th intercostal space on the lateral thorax (midline of the thorax), and above the 6th intercostal space on the anterior thorax (midline of the clavicle), perpendicular and deep insertion is prohibited to prevent injury to the heart and lungs. This is especially important for patients with emphysema to prevent pneumothorax.

c. The acupuncture points on the flanks and in the kidney area should not be perpendicularly or deeply needled to avoid injuring the liver, spleen, and kidneys. This is especially important for hepatomegaly and splenomegaly patients.

d. Attention must be paid to the angle and depth when needling the abdominal area of patients with gastric ulcers, intestinal adhesions, and intestinal obstruction, as well as the symphysis pubis of patients with urinary retention, as improper needling may lead to injury to the gastrointestinal tract and bladder.

e. Needling the acupuncture points located above the 1st lumbar vertebra along the midline of the nape and back should be approached with caution in terms of angle and depth, to avoid accidental injury to the medulla oblongata and spinal cord, which could have serious consequences. After needling these acupoints to a certain depth, if the patient experiences an electric shock sensation spreading to the limbs or the whole body, the needle should be immediately withdrawn.

Moxibustion Techniques

Moxibustion is often used in conjunction with acupuncture. It involves the application of moxa products (such as moxa sticks and moxa cones) as the primary material for therapeutic heat application. After ignition, these products are applied to acupuncture points or specific areas of the body to stimulate the body's meridian *qi* through the thermotherapeutic effect. This method helps adjust the functions of the *zang-fu* organs, thereby preventing and treating diseases.

Mugwort, a perennial semi-shrub herb of the Artemisia genus in the Asteraceae family with a strong fragrance, is widely used for moxibustion. With the exception of extremely arid and high-cold areas, mugwort can be found almost everywhere in China, and the mugwort produced in Qichun, Hubei Province in Central China, is considered the finest. As a traditional Chinese herb, it is known for its warming nature, fragrant aroma, and ability to regulate *qi* and blood, dispel cold and dampness, warm the meridians, and stop bleeding. Moxa wool made from mugwort has the advantage of being easily flammable and producing gentle heat, making it a preferred material for moxibustion.

The quality of moxa wool has a certain impact on the efficacy of moxibustion. Fresh moxa wool contains more volatile oils, leading to a stronger fire during moxibustion. On the other hand, aged moxa wool contains less volatile oil, resulting in a milder flame and better therapeutic effects. Moreover, substandard moxa wool exhibits higher impurity levels, lacks cohesion during combustion, and results in erratic flames, excessive smoke and a harsh odor. And its ash easily disperses, posing a risk of skin burns. In contrast, good-quality moxa wool has fewer impurities, produces less smoke and odor during burning, burns with a milder flame, and forms cohesive ash, minimizing scattering.

Common moxa products used in clinical practice include moxa cones and moxa sticks. There is a wide variety of moxa products available for purchase online, allowing users to choose according to their specific needs.

① Moxa cones. Place pure aged moxa wool on a flat surface, pinch and rotate with the thumb, index finger, and middle finger to form a cone-shaped mass, known as a moxa cone. Various molds for making moxa cones are available on the market, offering simplicity and convenience. Burning one moxa cone is referred to as one *zhuang*.

② Moxa sticks. They are cylindrical long rolls made by wrapping moxa wool with mulberry bark paper. There are numerous brands of moxa sticks available in different lengths and thicknesses to suit individual preferences. Moxa sticks can be classified as pure or medicated, depending on whether Chinese medicine powder is added to the moxa wool. Medicated moxa sticks often contain a blend of herbs such as cinnamon, dried ginger, clove, costus root, pubescent angelica root, asarum, radix angelicae, realgar, rhizoma atractylodis, myrrh, frankincense, and pericarpium zanthoxyli, finely ground and mixed into the moxa wool at a specific ratio of 6 grams per stick.

Common Moxibustion Methods

Common moxibustion methods in clinical practice include moxibustion with moxa cones, moxibustion with moxa sticks, moxibustion with a warming needle, and moxibustion with a moxibustioner.

★ Moxibustion with Moxa Cones

Moxibustion with moxa cones involves placing the cone on the skin over acupuncture points for treatment. This method can be categorized into direct and indirect moxibustion.

Direct moxibustion. The method entails applying the moxa cone directly onto the skin over acupuncture points. Due to the risk of burns, this method is less commonly used in clinical practice.

Indirect moxibustion. In this method, moxibustion is performed by placing certain substances, such as herbs, between the moxa cone and the skin over acupuncture points. This provides a dual effect of moxibustion and herbal therapy. Common indirect moxibustion methods include moxibustion with ginger, moxibustion with garlic, and moxibustion with salt.

① Moxibustion with ginger. Select suitable ginger segments and cut them into slices with a diameter of 2 to 3 cm and a thickness of 0.2 to 0.3 cm. Poke multiple small holes in the middle with a needle. Choose a suitable position and fully expose the acupuncture points that need moxibustion. Place the prepared ginger slices on the acupuncture points, and then place the moxa cone in the center of the ginger slices. Ignite the tip of the moxa cone to initiate burning. If the patient experiences unbearable local burning pain, briefly lift one side of the ginger slice using tweezers to alleviate discomfort before returning it and continuing with the moxibustion process. After the moxa cone burns out, remove the moxa ash and replace it with a new moxa cone for a new moxibustion sessions. If the ginger slices become burnt and withered, replace them with fresh ones. Generally, each acupuncture point is moxibusted 6 to 9 *zhuang* (moxa cones), until the local skin appears red but without blistering. This method is primarily used to treat superficies syndromes of exogenous disease and deficiency-cold diseases, such as colds, coughs, arthralgia caused by wind-cold-damp pathogens, vomiting, diarrhea, abdominal pain, etc.

② Moxibustion with garlic. Select single clove garlic, cut into slices 0.2 to 0.3 cm thick, and poke multiple small holes in the middle with a needle. The procedure of moxibustion with garlic closely resembles that of moxibustion with ginger, with 5 to 7 *zhuang* (moxa cones) at each acupuncture point. This moxibustion is known for its ability to reduce swelling, detoxify, alleviate pain, and disperse masses. It is commonly applied to treat conditions such as deep-seated ulceration with discharge, pale sore lacking redness or sensation, and non-suppurative ailments, unruptured carbuncles, and abscesses, as well as insect bites, snake bites, and stings from bees and scorpions.

③ Moxibustion with salt. Choose a suitable position and fully expose the acupuncture points that need moxibustion. Take an appropriate amount of clean and dry table salt and fill the umbilicus. In cases where the umbilicus is shallow, the salt may be elevated slightly above the skin to prevent burns. Optionally, a slice of ginger can be added on top of the salt. A moxa cone is ignited and placed on the salt (or ginger slice) to burn. If the patient finds the burning sensation unbearable, any remaining moxa cone should be removed and replaced with a new one. Repeat this process with 5 to 9 *zhuang* (moxa cones). This method has the therapeutic effects of restoring *yang*, rescuing collapse, and relieving depletion. It is commonly used for acute cold abdominal pain, vomiting and diarrhea, dysentery, dysuria, and apoplectic collapse.

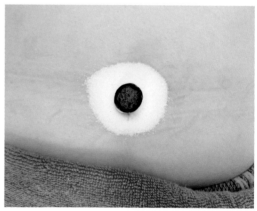

Fig. 1 Moxibustion with salt.

★ Moxibustion with Moxa Sticks

Moxibustion with moxa sticks involves applying moxibustion therapy using a burning moxa stick above the skin over acupuncture points. Common types of moxibustion with moxa sticks include mild-warm moxibustion, sparrow-pecking moxibustion, and revolving moxibustion.

① Mild-warm moxibustion. Choose a suitable position and fully expose the acupuncture points that need moxibustion. Ignite one end of the moxa stick and perform fumigation about 2 to 3 cm away from the skin at the acupuncture point, keeping the moxa stick relatively fixed with the moxibustion site. If the patient experiences excessive

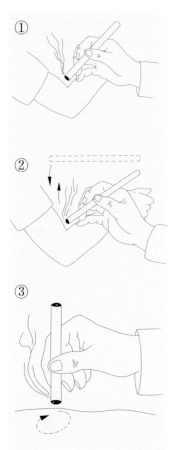

heat, adjust the distance between the moxa stick and the skin accordingly. The extent of moxibustion is determined by the appearance of local skin redness and warmth without any sensation of burning. Typically, each acupuncture point is treated with moxibustion for 5 to 15 minutes.

② Sparrow-pecking moxibustion. Ignite one end of the moxa stick and move it up and down in a manner reminiscent of a sparrow pecking at rice, varying the distance between the burning end of the moxa stick and the skin. Ensure a uniform speed and consistent rise and fall, and repeat the motion. Moxibustion should continue until the skin exhibits redness and warmth without any burning sensation, usually lasting for 5 to 15 minutes.

③ Revolving moxibustion. Ignite one end of the moxa stick and keep it at a relatively fixed distance from the moxibustion site, generally about 3 cm. Move it parallel or rotate it repeatedly at a uniform speed, and repeat the motion. Moxibustion should continue until the skin exhibits redness and warmth without any burning sensation, usually lasting for 5 to 15 minutes.

It is worth noting that during the process of moxibustion with moxa sticks, if treating children or patients with reduced skin sensation, the practitioner can place their index and middle fingers on either side of the treatment area to assess the patient's sensitivity to heat based on their fingertip sensations. This allows for timely adjustment of the distance to prevent burns.

⋆ Moxibustion with Warming Needle

This is a method that combines acupuncture and moxibustion, suitable for conditions that require both needle retention and moxibustion. Specific procedure is as follows: prepare several moxa sticks about 2 cm long, and make a small hole in the center of one end, about 1 to 1.5 cm deep.

Choose a suitable position and fully expose the acupuncture points that need moxibustion. Select a slightly thicker (generally 0.3 mm) acupuncture needle, insert it perpendicularly into the acupuncture point, and once the *qi* sensation is achieved, insert the end of the moxa stick with the hole onto the needle

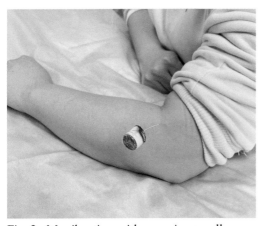

Fig. 2   Moxibustion with warming needle.

handle, and ignite the moxa stick. When the moxa stick burns out, remove the moxa ash into a container, replace it with a new segment of moxa stick, and apply 1 to 3 *zhuang* (moxa cones) of moxibustion per acupuncture point each time. Remove the needle after the needle handle is cooled.

★ Moxibustion with Moxibustioner

As people pay more attention to health, moxibustion therapy, as a natural treatment, is increasingly accepted by the public. The extensive use of moxibustion has led to the emergence of various moxibustioners. Commonly used moxibustioners are generally hollow inside, allowing moxa sticks to be inserted or placed within them, and they are widely available in the market. Moxibustion with a moxibustioner is relatively gentle and is often preferred by women, children, and those who fear moxibustion.

Moxibustion Sensation and Moxibustion Dosage

Moxibustion sensation refers to the special perception and response elicited in the human body during the moxibustion process, encompassing local and systemic sensations. This also includes observable changes after moxibustion, such as redness, sweating, muscle twitching, etc. There are several distinct sensations:

① Heat penetration. That is, the heat of moxibustion penetrates from the surface of the skin at the moxibustion site to the deeper tissues, sometimes reaching the thorax and abdomen organs. For instance, moxibusting the Shenque acupoint can produce a warming sensation throughout the abdomen, accompanied by increased gastrointestinal movement.

② Heat expansion. That is, the heat of moxibustion spreads from the moxibustion site to the surrounding area. For instance, moxibusting the Mingmen acupoint can cause heat to spread not only deep into tissues but also laterally to both sides of the waist.

③ Heat transfer. That is, the heat of moxibustion spreads from the moxibustion site to distal parts. For instance, moxibusting the Baliao point can conduct heat along the bladder meridian to the thighs, and even to the soles of the feet.

④ The area where moxibustion is applied may not feel heat or may only experience mild warmth, while areas distant from the moxibustion site feel warmer. For instance, moxibusting several acupuncture points along the small intestine meridian on the shoulder can result in warmth sensations in the arm and back.

⑤ The skin at the moxibustion site may not feel heat or may only experience mild warmth, while the deep tissues beneath the skin, and even the organs in the thorax and abdomen, feel warmer. For instance, moxibusting the Shenshu acupoint can result in warmth sensations in the abdomen and kidneys.

⑥ Moxibustion may also induce sensations such as soreness, numbness, swelling, pain, itching, cold, heat, wind, chill, cool, and muscle twitching, either at the moxibustion site or in distant areas, collectively known as heat-sensitive moxibustion sensations. For instance, moxibusting the Sanyinjiao acupoint may cause the feet to feel cold, as if a breeze is passing through and cool air is circulating between the toes.

Moxibustion dosage refers to the degree of thermal effect achieved during moxibustion. The moxibustion dosage is determined by the intensity of the moxibustion stimulation, the duration, and the frequency of moxibustion.

In general, the moxibustion dosage should be tailored to the patient's age, constitution, condition, and specific acupuncture point location to attain optimal results. For instance, young and robust patients in the early stages of illness benefit from a higher moxibustion dose, whereas elderly and frail individuals with chronic ailments require a lower dose. Areas with thicker flesh below the waist warrant a larger moxibustion dose, while those with shallow flesh in regions like the head, thorax, and limbs require a smaller dose. Patients exhibiting symptoms of depleted primordial *qi* and cold limbs benefit from a larger moxibustion dose, whereas those with conditions such as arthralgia caused by wind-cold-damp pathogens and excess in the upper part of the body and deficiency in the lower require a smaller dose. For chronic conditions, moxibustion can be administered every 2 to 3 days with a higher dose, whereas for acute cases, moxibustion can be applied 1 to 3 times daily with a lower dose.

Indications of Moxibustion

Modern research indicates that the near-infrared radiation emitted by burning moxa can be absorbed by the body, leading to an increase in deep subcutaneous temperature. This process promotes local blood and lymph circulation, enhances metabolism, and boosts the immune system by increasing the production of immunoglobulins and white blood cells while improving the phagocytic function of macrophages.

Furthermore, moxibustion serves as a preventive measure for diseases and contributes to health and longevity. It stimulates the body's vital *qi*, strengthening its ability to resist illnesses. Certain acupuncture points known for their reinforcing effects, such as Zhongwan, Guanyuan, Qihai, Mingmen, Shenshu, and Zusanli acupoints are commonly used for health moxibustion.

Clinically, moxibustion is usually applicable to the following conditions:

① Arthralgia caused by wind-cold-damp pathogens, dysmenorrhea, amenorrhea, and cold colic in the abdomen and vulva resulting from cold congealing blood stasis and blockade of meridians.

② Vomiting, abdominal pain, diarrhea, etc. resulting from superficies syndrome of exogenous wind-cold and deficient cold in middle *jiao*, as well as vomiting, chronic diarrhea, chronic dysentery, enuresis, menorrhagia, spermatorrhea, impotence, premature ejaculation, dizziness, anemia, amenorrhea, collapse, shock, etc. resulting from spleen-kidney *yang* deficiency, weak *qi* and blood, and excessive loss of vital *qi*.

③ Gastroptosis, nephroptosis, uterine prolapse, and rectal prolapse caused by deficiency and sinking of *qi* and visceroptosis.

④ Beriberi involving heart, and upward hyperactivity of liver *yang* resulting from adverse rising of *qi*.

⑤ Early-stage surgical ulcers, lymph node tuberculosis, etc.

⑥ Moxibustion can promote wound healing and tissue regeneration, particularly for long-term non-healing wounds or ulcers.

Contraindications of Moxibustion

① Moxibustion should follow a specific sequence, typically starting with the upper body before moving to the lower body, and addressing *yang* areas (such as the back and lateral limbs) before *yin* areas (including the thorax, abdomen, and medial limbs). The moxibustion sessions should gradually increase, and the size of moxa cones should start small and gradually enlarge. However, in special cases, moxibustion can be adjusted accordingly. For instance, in cases of rectal prolapse, moxibustion can be applied to the Changqiang acupoint to contract the anus, followed by the Baihui acupoint to lift the prolapse.

② Avoid moxibustion on areas with thin skin, less flesh, tendon-muscle convergence, great vessels, the precordial region, the lumbosacral and lower abdominal areas of pregnant women, the nipple area, the genital area, and the testicles.

③ Moxibustion is not suitable for individuals experiencing extreme fatigue, excessive hunger or fullness, intoxication, profuse sweating, emotional instability, fear of moxibustion, menstruating women, acute infectious diseases, high fever, coma, seizures, extreme emaciation and exhaustion, or mental illness. Moxibustion should only be performed once these conditions have been resolved.

④ Moxibustion is generally not suitable for individuals with symptoms of excessive heat syndrome and *yin* deficiency, such as hypertensive crisis, advanced pulmonary tuberculosis, massive hemoptysis, vomiting, severe anemia, acute infectious diseases, and skin carbuncle-abscess and furunculosis with fever.

⑤ If blisters appear after moxibustion: for small blisters, avoid puncturing them and let them absorb naturally; for large blisters, use a sterilized fine needle to puncture the edge of the blister parallel to the skin, release the fluid, or use a syringe to extract the fluid, then disinfect with iodine and wrap with gauze. If the blister pus turns yellow-green or shows signs of oozing blood due to improper care and infection, prompt medical attention should be sought. In cases of prolonged moxibustion leading to dry mouth and thirst, the patient can slowly drink warm water.

CHAPTER FOUR

Acupuncture Treatment for Internal Conditions

This chapter covers common internal conditions such as colds, stomachaches, headaches, constipation, and insomnia. Note that acupuncture should be performed by professionals. Please exercise caution, ensuring that the intensity of acupuncture is within the patient's comfort level.

Colds

A cold is a prevalent exogenous ailment characterized by symptoms such as nasal obstruction, runny nose, aversion to cold with fever, cough, headache, and overall discomfort. It can occur year-round but is more common in winter and spring, primarily due to exposure to wind pathogens. The pathological focus of this condition is on the lungs, and acupuncture is employed to dispel wind and relieve superficies.

The main acupuncture points include Lieque, Hegu, Fengchi, and Dazhui. Specific acupuncture points for different patterns are as follows:

Patterns	Diagnostic Features	Acupuncture Points
Wind-cold syndrome	Severe aversion to cold, mild fever, soreness and pain in the limbs, thin and white phlegm, thin and white tongue coating	Main acupoints + Waiguan, Fengmen, Feishu
Wind-heat syndrome	Severe fever, mild aversion to cold, yellow and sticky phlegm, thin and yellow tongue coating	Main acupoints + Quchi, Chize
Summerheat-dampness syndrome	Inefficient perspiration, heavy and throbbing headache, nausea and discomfort, loose stools, thin and yellow greasy tongue coating	Main acupoints + Zusanli, Zhongwan

Procedure: Conventional needle insertion. Specific procedures can be found below for each acupuncture point. (Simplified as "conventional needle insertion" in the ensuing text.)

Position: Lateral position.

Main Acupoints

1. Lieque Acupoint

Location: Cross the hands naturally with the tiger's mouth (fleshy part of the hand in the

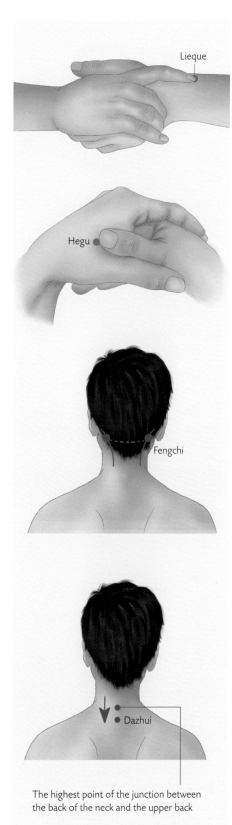

Lieque

Hegu

Fengchi

Dazhui

The highest point of the junction between the back of the neck and the upper back

junction between the thumb and index finger is called the tiger's mouth), and press one index finger on the styloid process of the radius (the high prominence on the thumb side behind the wrist). The acupuncture point is located under the fingertip of the index finger.

Procedure: Insert the needle perpendicularly or obliquely into a depth of 0.5 to 1 cun, retaining it for 20 to 30 minutes.

2. Hegu Acupoint

Location: On the back of the hand, between the 1st and 2nd metacarpal bones, at the midpoint of the radial side on the 2nd metacarpal bone.

Quick location: Take the crease of the thumb interphalangeal joint of one hand and place it on the edge of the web between the thumb and forefinger of the other hand, where the tip of the thumb lands is Hegu acupoint.

Procedure: Insert the needle perpendicularly or obliquely into a depth of 0.5 to 1 cun, retaining it for 20 to 30 minutes.

3. Fengchi Acupoint

Location: In the posterior neck region, below the occipital bone, in the depression between the upper end of the sternocleidomastoid muscle and the trapezius muscle.

Quick location: Sit upright, and the acupoint is situated in the depression on the lateral edge of the two major tendons below the occipital bone, level with the earlobe.

Procedure: Insert the needle obliquely towards the tip of the nose with the tips of the needle slightly downwards, into a depth of 0.5 to 0.8 cun, or insert the needle horizontally towards the Fengfu acupoint (see page 133), retaining it for 20 to 30 minutes.

4. Dazhui Acupoint

Location: In the spinal area, below the spinous process of the 7th cervical vertebra, on the posterior midline.

Quick location: Lower the head, and

the highest point of the junction between the back of the neck and the upper back corresponds to the spinous process of the 7th cervical vertebra, and the depression below it is the Dazhui acupoint.

Procedure: Insert the needle perpendicularly or obliquely into a depth of 0.5 to 1 cun, retaining it for 20 to 30 minutes.

Wind-Cold Syndrome: Main Acupoints + Waiguan, Fengmen, Shenshu

1. Waiguan Acupoint

Location: One the posterior antebrachial area, 2 cun (3-finger width) above the dorsal wrist crease, on the midpoint of the gap between the ulna and radius (two major bones).

Procedure: Insert the needle perpendicularly or obliquely into a depth of 0.5 to 1 cun, retaining it for 20 to 30 minutes.

2. Fengmen Acupoint

Location: On the back, below the spinous process of the 2nd thoracic vertebra, 1.5 cun lateral to the posterior midline.

Quick location: Lower the head, and the highest point of the junction between the back of the neck and the upper back corresponds to the spinous process of the 7th cervical vertebra. Count down 2 vertebrae, the acupoint is situated 2-finger width beside the lower edge.

Procedure: Insert the needle obliquely into a depth of 0.5 to 0.8 cun, avoiding deep insertion to prevent visceral organ injury, and retaining it for 20 to 30 minutes.

3. Feishu Acupoint

Location: On the back, below the spinous process of the 3rd thoracic vertebra, 1.5 cun lateral to the posterior midline.

Quick location: Lower the head, and the highest point of the junction between the back of the neck and the upper back corresponds to the spinous process of the 7th cervical vertebra. Count down 3 vertebrae, the acupoint is situated 2-finger width beside the lower edge.

Procedure: Insert the needle obliquely into a depth of 0.5 to 0.8 cun, avoiding deep and

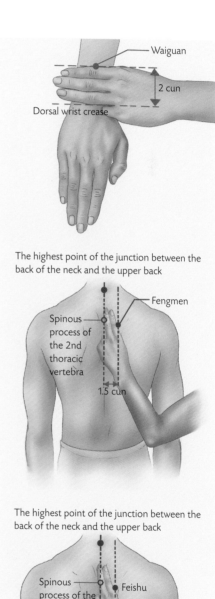

Waiguan

2 cun

Dorsal wrist crease

The highest point of the junction between the back of the neck and the upper back

Fengmen

Spinous process of the 2nd thoracic vertebra

1.5 cun

The highest point of the junction between the back of the neck and the upper back

Spinous process of the 3rd thoracic vertebra

Feishu

1.5 cun

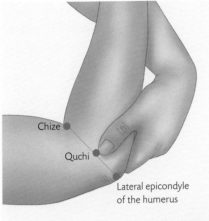

Chize

Quchi

Lateral epicondyle
of the humerus

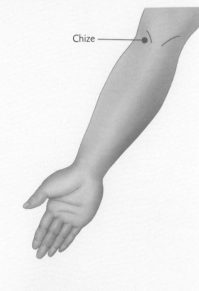

Chize

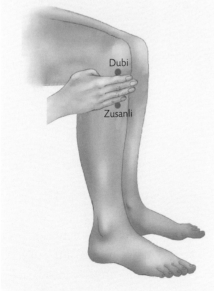

Dubi

Zusanli

perpendicular insertion to prevent visceral organ injury, and retaining it for 20 to 30 minutes.

Wind-Heat Syndrome: Main Acupoints + Quchi, Chize

1. Quchi Acupoint

Location: At the lateral end of the cubital crease, with the elbow flexed, at the midpoint of the line connecting the Chize acupoint with the lateral epicondyle of the humerus.

Procedure: Insert the needle perpendicularly or obliquely into a depth of 0.5 to 1 cun, retaining it for 20 to 30 minutes.

2. Chize Acupoint

Location: In the depression on the radial side of the biceps brachii tendon in the cubital crease.

Quick location: With the palm facing up and the elbow slightly bent, locate the large tendon (biceps brachii tendon) in the middle of the elbow. The acupoint is situated in the depression on the lateral aspect (thumb side) of the cubital crease.

Procedure: Insert the needle perpendicularly or obliquely into a depth of 0.5 to 1 cun, retaining it for 20 to 30 minutes.

Summerheat-Dampness Syndrome: Main Acupoints + Zusanli, Zhongwan

1. Zusanli Acupoint

Location: On the front lateral aspect of the lower leg, 3 cun (about 4-finger width) below the Dubi acupoint, 1-finger width lateral to the anterior crest of the tibia.

Quick location: Stand and bend over; use the tiger's mouth of hand on the same side to encircle the upper outer edge of the patella, with the remaining 4 fingers pointing downward, and the tip of the middle finger is this acupoint.

Procedure: Insert the needle perpendicularly or obliquely into a depth of 0.5 to 1 cun, retaining it for 20 to 30 minutes.

2. Zhongwan Acupoint

Location: In the upper abdomen, at the midpoint of the line connecting the xiphisternal symphysis with the umbilicus.

Procedure: Insert the needle perpendicularly or obliquely into a depth of 0.5 to 1 cun, retaining it for 20 to 30 minutes.

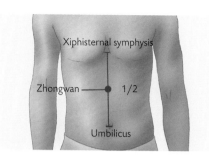

 Physician's advice: ① Acupuncture treatment has better effects on colds. If the patient's symptoms worsen, consider comprehensive treatment. ② Ensure proper room ventilation.

Cough

Cough is characterized by impaired diffusion, purification, and descending of lung *qi*, sounds due to the upward counterflowing of lung *qi*, and the expectoration of sputum. It stands as a primary symptom of lung disorders, often manifesting as audible coughing or coughing accompanied by sputum. Exogenous cough is caused by the invasion of six climatic exopathogens into the lungs; endogenous cough is caused by the dysfunction of the *zang-fu* organs accumulating in the lungs. The pathological focus of this condition is on the lungs. Acupuncture treatment focuses on regulating lung function and alleviating cough.

Specific acupuncture points for different patterns are as follows:

Patterns	Diagnostic Features	Acupuncture Points
Exogenous cough	Thin white or sticky yellow phlegm, aversion to cold and fever	Feishu, Lieque, Hegu
Endogenous cough	Cough caused by no external pathogenic factors	Feishu, Taiyuan, Danzhong

Procedure: Conventional needle insertion.
Position: Sitting position.

Exogenous Cough

1. Feishu Acupoint

Location: On the back, below the spinous process of the 3rd thoracic vertebra, 1.5 cun lateral to the posterior midline.

Quick location: Lower the head, and the highest point of the junction between the back of the neck and the upper back corresponds to the spinous process of the 7th cervical vertebra. Count down 3 vertebrae, the acupoint is situated 2-finger width beside the lower edge.

The highest point of the junction between the back of the neck and the upper back

Spinous process of the 3rd thoracic vertebra

Feishu

1.5 cun

Lieque

Hegu

The highest point of the junction between the back of the neck and the upper back

Spinous process of the 3rd thoracic vertebra

Feishu

1.5 cun

Procedure: Avoid perpendicular and deep needle insertion on the Feishu acupoint to prevent visceral organ injury. Utilize the twirling reducing method and insert the needle obliquely into a depth of 0.5 to 0.8 cun, retaining it for 20 to 30 minutes.

2. Lieque Acupoint

Location: Cross the hands naturally with the tiger's mouth, and press one index finger on the styloid process of the radius (the high prominence on the thumb side behind the wrist). The acupuncture point is located under the fingertip of the index finger.

Procedure: Utilize the reducing methods by lifting-thrusting or twirling, and insert the needle perpendicularly or obliquely into a depth of 0.5 to 1 cun, retaining it for 20 to 30 minutes.

3. Hegu Acupoint

Location: On the back of the hand, between the 1st and 2nd metacarpal bones, at the midpoint of the radial side on the 2nd metacarpal bone.

Quick location: Take the crease of the thumb interphalangeal joint of one hand and place it on the edge of the web between the thumb and forefinger of the other hand, where the tip of the thumb lands is Hegu acupoint.

Procedure: Utilize the reducing method, and insert the needle perpendicularly or obliquely into a depth of 0.5 to 1 cun, retaining it for 20 to 30 minutes.

Endogenous Cough

1. Feishu Acupoint

Location: On the back, below the spinous process of the 3rd thoracic vertebra, 1.5 cun lateral to the posterior midline.

Quick location: Lower the head, and the highest point of the junction between the back of the neck and the upper back corresponds to the spinous process of the 7th cervical vertebra. Count down 3 vertebrae, the point is situated

2-finger width beside the lower edge.

Procedure: Avoid perpendicular and deep needle insertion on the Feishu acupoint to prevent visceral organ injury. Utilize the even reinforcing-reducing method or twirling reinforcing method and insert the needle obliquely into a depth of 0.5 to 0.8 cun, retaining it for 20 to 30 minutes.

2. Taiyuan Acupoint

Location: On the palmar wrist crease on the radial side, precisely at the point of pulsation of the radial artery.

Procedure: Caution must be exercised to avoid the radial artery during needle insertion. Utilize the even reinforcing-reducing method or twirling reinforcing method, and insert the needle perpendicularly into a depth of 0.3 cun, retaining it for 20 to 30 minutes.

3. Danzhong Acupoint

Location: In the thorax, at the midpoint between the nipples, horizontally at the 4th intercostal space.

Procedure: Employ skin-pinching up needle inserting method, and insert the needle horizontally into a depth of 0.3 to 0.5 cun, retaining it for 20 to 30 minutes.

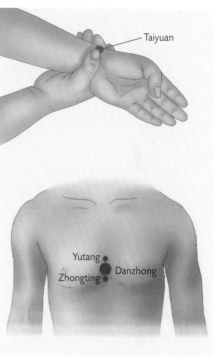

 Physician's advice: ① Acupuncture is more effective in the early stage of this condition. ② Actively engage in cardiovascular and pulmonary exercise to improve immune function. ③ Quitting smoking is of great significance for the recovery of this condition.

Asthma

Asthma is a paroxysmal respiratory condition characterized by sputum wheezing and difficulty breathing. During an attack, there is rapid breathing, wheezing in the throat, and in severe cases, mouth breathing with shoulder elevation and flaring of the nostrils, making it difficult to lie flat. This condition can attack recurrently and occur at any age and season, especially during cold seasons and sudden climate changes. The pathological focus of this condition is on the lungs. Acupuncture treatment focuses on relieving wheezing and breathing difficulties.

The main acupuncture points include Feishu, Taiyuan, Dingchuan, and Danzhong. Specific acupuncture points for different patterns are as follows:

Patterns	Diagnostic Features	Acupuncture Points
Excess syndrome	Short duration of the disease, high-pitched and coarse wheezing, deep and long breaths in excess, with the main manifestation of deep exhalation, and thin tongue coating	Main acupoints + Chize, Yuji
Deficiency syndrome	Long duration of the disease, low-pitched and timid wheezing, tendency for severe wheezing with movement and shortness of breath, with the main manifestation of deep inhalation, and pale tongue	Main acupoints + Shenshu

Procedure: Conventional needle insertion.

Position: Sitting position.

Main Acupoints

1. Feishu Acupoint

Location: On the back, below the spinous process of the 3rd thoracic vertebra, 1.5 cun lateral to the posterior midline.

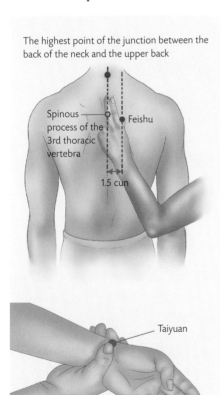

The highest point of the junction between the back of the neck and the upper back

Spinous process of the 3rd thoracic vertebra

Feishu

1.5 cun

Taiyuan

Quick location: Lower the head, and the highest point of the junction between the back of the neck and the upper back corresponds to the spinous process of the 7th cervical vertebra. Count down 3 vertebrae, the point is situated 2-finger width beside the lower edge.

Procedure: Avoid perpendicular and deep needle insertion on the Feishu acupoint to prevent visceral organ injury. Insert the needle obliquely into a depth of 0.5 to 0.8 cun, retaining it for 20 to 30 minutes.

2. Taiyuan Acupoint

Location: On the palmar wrist crease on the radial side, precisely at the point of pulsation of the radial artery.

Procedure: Caution must be exercised to avoid the radial artery during needle insertion. Insert the needle perpendicularly into a depth of 0.3 cun, retaining it for 20 to 30 minutes.

3. Dingchuan Acupoint

Location: On the back, below the spinous process of the 7th cervical vertebra, 0.5 cun lateral to the posterior midline.

Quick location: Lower the head, and the highest point of the junction between the back of the neck and the upper back corresponds to the spinous process of the 7th cervical vertebra. The acupoint is situated below, half-finger width lateral to the Dazhui acupoint.

Procedure: Insert the needle perpendicularly or obliquely into a depth of 0.5 to 1 cun, retaining it for 20 to 30 minutes.

4. Danzhong Acupoint

Location: In the thorax, at the midpoint between the nipples, horizontally at the 4th intercostal space.

Procedure: Employ skin-pinching up needle inserting method, and insert the needle horizontally into a depth of 0.3 to 0.5 cun, retaining it for 20 to 30 minutes.

Excess Syndrome: Main Acupoints + Chize, Yuji

1. Chize Acupoint

Location: In the depression on the radial side of the biceps brachii tendon in the cubital crease.

Quick location: With the palm facing up and the elbow slightly bent, locate the large tendon (biceps brachii tendon) in the middle of the elbow. The point is situated in the depression on the lateral aspect (thumb side) of the cubital crease.

Procedure: Insert the needle perpendicularly or obliquely into a depth of 0.5 to 1 cun , retaining it for 20 to 30 minutes.

2. Yuji Acupoint

Location: Posterior to the 1st metacarpophalangeal joint, at the junction of the red and white flesh on the radial side of the midpoint of the 1st metacarpal bone.

Procedure: Insert the needle perpendicularly or obliquely into a depth of 0.5 to 1 cun, retaining it for 20 to 30 minutes.

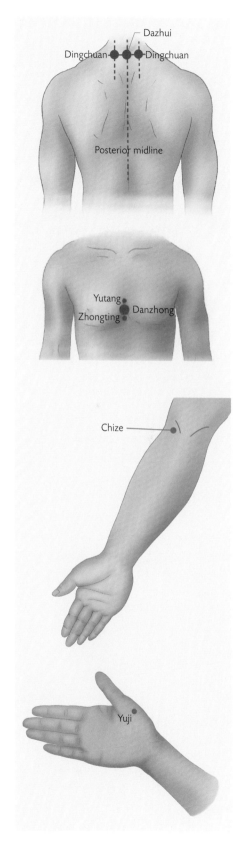

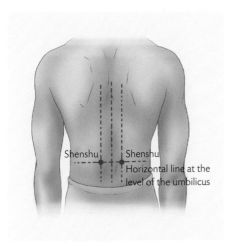

Deficiency Syndrome: Main Acupoints +
Shenshu Acupoint

Shenshu Acupoint

Location: In the lumbar region, below the spinous process of the 2nd lumbar vertebra, 1.5 cun lateral to the posterior midline.

Quick location: 2-finger width lateral to the intersection of the horizontal line at the level of the umbilicus and the spine.

Procedure: Insert the needle perpendicularly or obliquely into a depth of 0.5 to 1 cun, retaining it for 20 to 30 minutes.

Physician's advice: ① Asthma often coexists with multiple conditions and necessitates proactive management of underlying diseases. ② Allergic asthma patients should steer clear of allergens.

Stroke

Stroke is characterized by sudden loss of consciousness, accompanied by facial asymmetry, speech impairment, and hemiplegia. The pathological focus of this condition is on the brain. In the acute phase, acupuncture is employed to awaken the brain and clear the meridians, while in the recovery phase, it focuses on clearing the meridians and harmonizing *qi* and blood.

According to the clinical stages of the acute phase and recovery phase, the acupuncture points are selected as follows:

Clinical Stages	Diagnostic Features	Acupuncture Points
Acute phase	Hemiplegia, language impairment, facial asymmetry with consciousness disorders	Shuigou, Neiguan, Jiquan, Chize, Weizhong, Sanyinjiao
Recovery phase	Gradual improvement of consciousness, with main focus on physical functional impairment	Main acupoints: Baihui, Fengchi, Shousanli, Hegu, Zusanli, Chize, Neiguan, Daling, Xuehai, Yinlingquan, Sanyinjiao, Taichong
		Facial asymmetry: Main acupoints + Dicang, Jiache Aphasia: Main acupoints + Yamen, Lianquan Drooling: Main acupoints + Chengjiang

Procedure: Conventional needle insertion.
Position: Lateral position.

Acute Phase

1. Shuigou Acupoint

Location: On the face, at the upper trisection point of the philtrum groove.

Procedure: Insert the needle obliquely upward into a depth of 0.3 to 0.5 cun, then perform shallow and quick lifting and thrusting method at the acupoint.

2. Neiguan Acupoint

Location: On the palmar aspect of the forearm, 2 cun above the palmar wrist crease, between the palmaris longus tendon and the flexor carpi radialis tendon.

Quick location: 3-finger width above the palmar wrist crease, between the two major tendons.

Procedure: Utilize the twirling reducing method, and insert the needle perpendicularly into a depth of 0.5 to 1 cun, retaining it for 20 to 30 minutes.

3. Jiquan Acupoint

Location: On the outer extension of the upper arm, at the apex of the armpit, where the axillary artery pulsates.

Procedure: Utilize the lifting-thrusting reducing method, and insert the needle perpendicularly into a depth of 0.5 to1 cun. The degree is determined by the presence of numbness, distension, and twitching in the upper limb. Retain the needle for 20 to 30 minutes.

4. Chize Acupoint

Location: In the depression on the radial side of the biceps brachii tendon in the cubital crease.

Quick location: With the palm facing up and the elbow slightly bent, locate the large tendon (biceps brachii tendon) in the middle of the elbow. The point is situated in the depression on the lateral aspect (thumb side) of the cubital crease.

Procedure: Utilize the lifting-thrusting

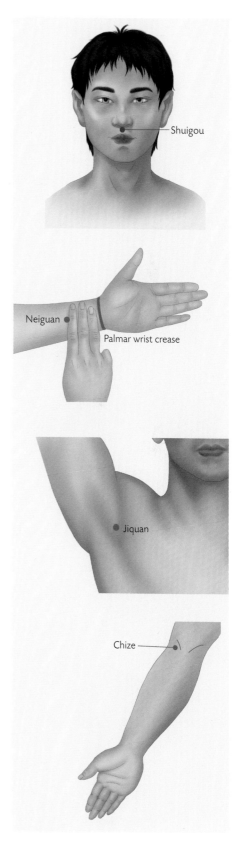

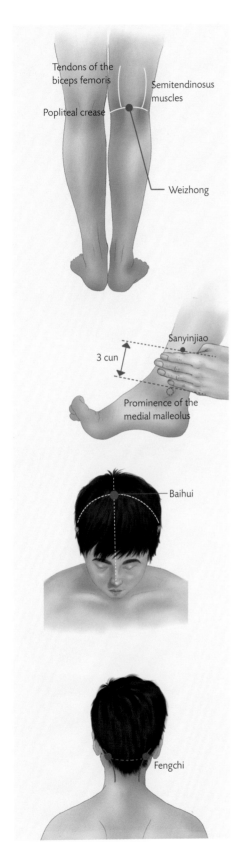

Tendons of the biceps femoris

Semitendinosus muscles

Popliteal crease

Weizhong

3 cun

Sanyinjiao

Prominence of the medial malleolus

Baihui

Fengchi

reducing method, and insert the needle perpendicularly into a depth of 0.5 to 1 cun, inducing limb twitching; retain the needle for 20 to 30 minutes.

5. Weizhong Acupoint

Location: In the posterior knee area, at the midpoint of the popliteal crease, between the tendons of the biceps femoris and semitendinosus muscles.

Procedure: Utilize the lifting-thrusting reducing method, and insert the needle perpendicularly into a depth of 1 to 1.5 cun inducing limb twitching; retain the needle for 20 to 30 minutes.

6. Sanyinjiao Acupoint

Location: On the medial aspect of the lower leg, 3 cun (4-finger width) above the prominence of the medial malleolus, posterior to the medial border of the tibia.

Procedure: Utilize the lifting-thrusting reinforcing method, and insert the needle perpendicularly or obliquely into a depth of 0.5 to 1 cun; retain the needle for 20 to 30 minutes.

Recovery Phase

1. Baihui Acupoint

Location: On the head, at the intersection of the line connecting both ear tips and the midline of the head.

Procedure: Insert the needle horizontally into a depth of 0.5 to 0.8 cun, retaining it for 20 to 30 minutes.

2. Fengchi Acupoint

Location: In the posterior neck region, below the occipital bone, in the depression between the upper end of the sternocleidomastoid muscle and the trapezius muscle.

Quick location: Sit upright, and the acupoint is situated in the depression on the lateral edge of the two major tendons below the occipital bone, level with the earlobe.

Procedure: Insert the needle obliquely towards the tip of the nose with the tips of the needle slightly downwards, into a depth of 0.5 to 0.8 cun, or insert the needle horizontally towards the Fengfu acupoint (see page 133), retaining it for 20 to 30 minutes.

3. Shousanli Acupoint

Location: On the lateral aspect of the dorsum of the forearm, along the line connecting Yangxi acupoint and Quchi acupoint, 2 cun (3-finger width) below the cubital crease.

Procedure: Insert the needle perpendicularly into a depth of 0.5 to 1.2 cun, retaining it for 20 to 30 minutes.

4. Hegu Acupoint

Location: On the back of the hand, between the 1st and 2nd metacarpal bones, at the midpoint of the radial side on the 2nd metacarpal bone.

Quick location: Take the crease of the thumb interphalangeal joint of one hand and place it on the edge of the web between the thumb and forefinger of the other hand, where the tip of the thumb lands is Hegu acupoint.

Procedure: Insert the needle perpendicularly or obliquely into a depth of 0.5 to 1 cun, retaining it for 20 to 30 minutes.

5. Zusanli Acupoint

Location: On the front lateral aspect of the lower leg, 3 cun (about 4-finger width) below the Dubi acupoint, 1-finger width lateral to the anterior crest of the tibia.

Quick location: Stand and bend over; use the tiger's mouth of hand on the same side to encircle the upper outer edge of the patella, with the remaining 4 fingers pointing downward, and the tip of the middle finger is this point.

Procedure: Insert the needle perpendicularly or obliquely into a depth of 0.5 to 1 cun, retaining it for 20 to 30 minutes.

6. Chize Acupoint

Location: In the depression on the radial

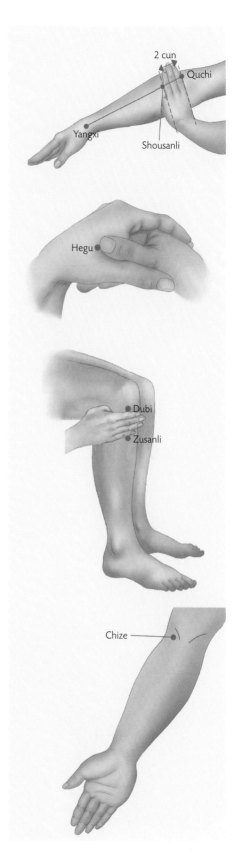

side of the biceps brachii tendon in the cubital crease.

Quick location: With the palm facing up and the elbow slightly bent, locate the large tendon (biceps brachii tendon) in the middle of the elbow. The point is situated in the depression on the lateral aspect (thumb side) of the cubital crease.

Procedure: Insert the needle perpendicularly or obliquely into a depth of 0.5 to 1 cun, retaining it for 20 to 30 minutes.

7. Neiguan Acupoint

Location: On the palmar aspect of the forearm, 2 cun above the palmar wrist crease, between the palmaris longus tendon and the flexor carpi radialis tendon.

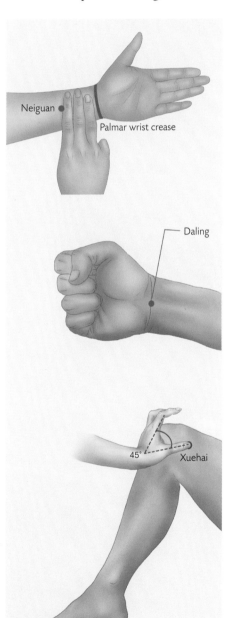

Quick location: 3-finger width above the palmar wrist crease, between the two major tendons.

Procedure: Utilize the twirling reducing method, and insert the needle perpendicularly into a depth of 0.5 to 1 cun, retaining it for 20 to 30 minutes.

8. Daling Acupoint

Location: At the midpoint of the palmar wrist crease, between the palmaris longus tendon and the flexor carpi radialis tendon.

Quick location: Slightly flex the wrist and make a fist, and the point is located on the palmar wrist crease, between the two major tendons.

Procedure: Insert the needle perpendicularly into a depth of 0.3 to 0.5 cun, retaining it for 20 to 30 minutes.

9. Xuehai Acupoint

Location: Bend the knee; on the medial aspect of the thigh, 2 cun above the medial end of the base of the patella, at the medial prominence of the quadriceps femoris muscle.

Quick location: Place the left (right) palm directly above the upper edge of the right (left) knee pan on the inner side of the thigh. Extend the 2nd to 5th fingers upward in a straight line, while maintaining a 45° angle between the thumb and the other four fingers. The acupoint is just beneath the tip of the thumb.

Procedure: Insert the needle perpendicularly into a depth of 1 to 1.5 cun, retaining it for 20 to 30 minutes.

10. Yinlingquan Acupoint

Location: On the medial aspect of the lower leg, in the depression below the posterior aspect of the medial malleolus of the tibia.

Quick location: Use the index finger to move upward along the medial aspect of the lower leg, reaching the depression where the tibia bends inward and upward, just below the knee joint.

Procedure: Insert the needle perpendicularly or obliquely into a depth of 1.5 to 2 cun, retaining it for 20 to 30 minutes.

11. Sanyinjiao Acupoint

Location: On the medial aspect of the lower leg, 3 cun (4-finger width) above the prominence of the medial malleolus, posterior to the medial border of the tibia.

Procedure: Utilize the lifting-thrusting reinforcing method, and insert the needle perpendicularly or obliquely into a depth of 0.5 to 1 cun; retain the needle for 20 to 30 minutes.

12. Taichong Acupoint

Location: On the dorsum of the foot, in the depression in front of the junction between the 1st and 2nd metatarsal bones.

Quick location: On the dorsum of the foot, push upward along the crease between the 1st and 2nd toes. The depression felt is the Taichong acupoint.

Procedure: Insert the needle perpendicularly or obliquely into a depth of 0.5 to 1 cun, retaining it for 20 to 30 minutes.

13. Dicang Acupoint

Location: On the face, lateral to the corner of the mouth, directly below the pupil.

Procedure: Insert the needle horizontally towards the direction of Jiache acupoint (see page 62) into a depth of 0.5 to 0.8 cun, retaining it for 20 to 30 minutes.

14. Jiache Acupoint

Location: On the face, in the depression when the masseter muscle bulges during

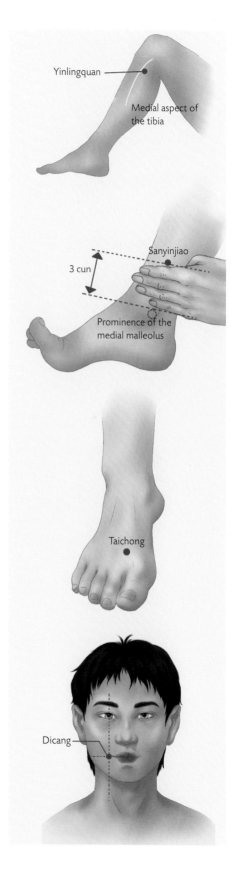

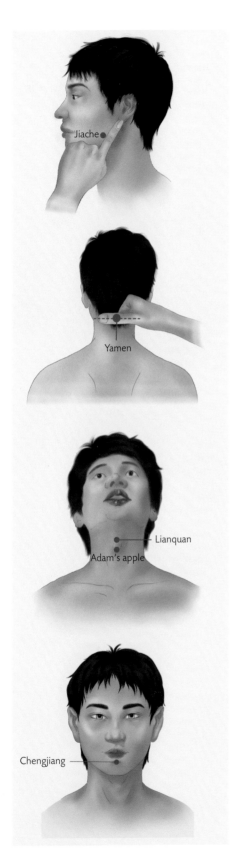

chewing.

Quick location: On the face, 1-finger width (middle finger) above the anterior superior angle of the mandible.

Procedure: Insert the needle perpendicularly into a depth of 0.3 to 0.5 cun, or insert the needle horizontally into a depth of 1 to 1.5 cun towards the direction of Dicang acupoint (see page 61), retaining it for 20 to 30 minutes.

15. Yamen Acupoint

Location: On the nape, 0.5 cun (half-finger width) directly above the midpoint of the posterior hairline, below the 1st cervical vertebra.

Procedure: Slowly insert the needle in a downward direction towards the lower mandible into a depth of 0.5 to 1 cun, avoiding upward insertion and retaining the needle for 20 to 30 minutes.

16. Lianquan Acupoint

Location: On the neck, along the anterior midline, above the Adam's apple, in the depression on the upper edge of the hyoid bone.

Procedure: Insert the needle horizontally towards the root of the tongue into a depth of 0.5 to 0.8 cun, retaining it for 20 to 30 minutes.

17. Chengjiang Acupoint

Location: On the face, in the middle depression of the mentolabial sulcus.

Procedure: Insert the needle obliquely into a depth of 0.3 to 0.5 cun, retaining it for 20 to 30 minutes.

> **Physician's advice:**
> ① Acupuncture demonstrates better therapeutic effects in treating strokes, especially in the rehabilitation of neurological function. ② Stroke patients should pay attention to the prevention and treatment of pressure sores and ensure unobstructed breathing.

Vertigo

Vertigo is a pathological condition characterized by dizziness and visual spinning. The pathological focus of this condition is on the brain. During acupuncture treatment, it is essential to conduct relevant examinations simultaneously to ascertain the underlying cause.

Specific acupuncture points for different patterns are as follows:

Patterns	Diagnostic Features	Acupuncture Points
Excess syndrome	Dizziness with tinnitus, irritability, or stuffiness in the head, greasy and white tongue coating, or dizziness with headache, dark tongue with stasis spots	Baihui, Fengchi, Taichong, Neiguan, Fenglong
Deficiency syndrome	Prolonged dizziness, fatigue, lack of sleep, forgetfulness, pale tongue with a thin coating	Baihui, Fengchi, Shenshu, Ganshu, Zusanli

Procedure: Conventional needle insertion.

Position: Prone position or lateral position.

Excess Syndrome

1. Baihui Acupoint

Location: On the head, at the intersection of the line connecting both ear tips and the midline of the head.

Procedure: Insert the needle horizontally into a depth of 0.5 to 0.8 cun, retaining it for 20 to 30 minutes.

2. Fengchi Acupoint

Location: In the posterior neck region, below the occipital bone, in the depression between the upper end of the sternocleidomastoid muscle and the trapezius muscle.

Quick location: Sit upright, and the acupoint is situated in the depression on the lateral edge of the two major tendons below the occipital bone, level with the earlobe.

Procedure: Insert the needle obliquely towards the tip of the nose with the tip of the needle slightly downward, into a depth of 0.5 to 0.8 cun, or insert the needle horizontally towards the Fengfu acupoint (see page 133), retaining it for 20 to 30 minutes.

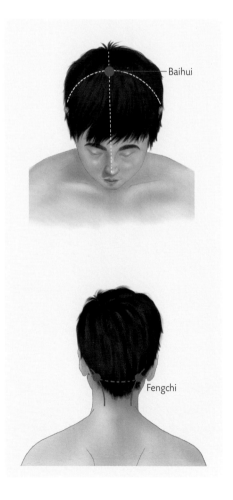

Baihui

Fengchi

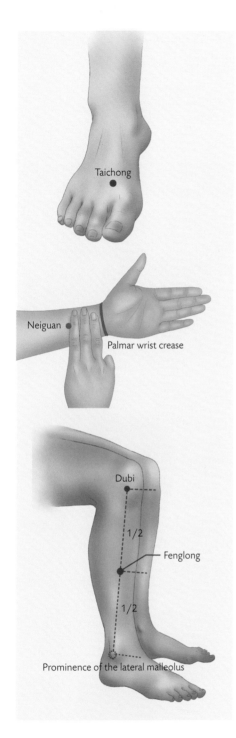

3. Taichong Acupoint

Location: On the dorsum of the foot, in the depression in front of the junction between the 1st and 2nd metatarsal bones.

Quick location: On the dorsum of the foot, push upward along the crease between the 1st and 2nd toes. The depression felt is the Taichong acupoint.

Procedure: Insert the needle perpendicularly or obliquely into a depth of 0.5 to 1 cun, retaining it for 20 to 30 minutes.

4. Neiguan Acupoint

Location: On the palmar aspect of the forearm, along the line connecting the Quze acupoint and the Daling acupoint, 2 cun above the palmar wrist crease, between the palmaris longus tendon and the flexor carpi radialis tendon.

Quick location: 3-finger width above the palmar wrist crease, between the two major tendons.

Procedure: Insert the needle perpendicularly or obliquely into a depth of 0.5 to 1 cun, retaining it for 20 to 30 minutes.

5. Fenglong Acupoint

Location: On the front lateral aspect of the lower leg, 8 cun above the prominence of the lateral malleolus, 2-finger width from the anterior edge of the tibia.

Quick location: Bend the knee, draw a line between Dubi acupoint and the prominence of the lateral malleolus, and find it at the midpoint of the line.

Procedure: Insert the needle perpendicularly or obliquely into a depth of 0.5 to 1 cun, retaining it for 20 to 30 minutes.

Deficiency Syndrome

1. Baihui Acupoint

Location: On the head, at the intersection of the line connecting both ear tips and the midline of the head.

Procedure: Insert the needle horizontally into a depth of 0.5 to 0.8 cun, retaining it for 20 to 30 minutes.

2. Fengchi Acupoint

Location: In the posterior neck region, below the occipital bone, in the depression between the upper end of the sternocleidomastoid muscle and the trapezius muscle.

Quick location: Sit upright, and the acupoint is situated in the depression on the lateral edge of the two major tendons below the occipital bone, level with the earlobe.

Procedure: Insert the needle obliquely towards the tip of the nose with the tip of the needle slightly downward, into a depth of 0.5 to 0.8 cun, or insert the needle horizontally towards the Fengfu acupoint (see page 133), retaining it for 20 to 30 minutes.

3. Shenshu Acupoint

Location: In the lumbar region, in the depression below the spinous process of the 2nd lumbar vertebra, 1.5 cun lateral to the posterior midline.

Quick location: 2-finger width lateral to the intersection of the horizontal line at the level of the umbilicus and the spine.

Procedure: Insert the needle perpendicularly or obliquely into a depth of 0.5 to 1 cun, retaining it for 20 to 30 minutes.

4. Ganshu Acupoint

Location: On the back, in the depression below the spinous process of the 9th thoracic vertebra, 1.5 cun lateral to the posterior midline.

Quick location: 2 vertebrae below the intersection of the horizontal line drawn from the inferior angle of the scapula and the spine (the spinous process of the 7th thoracic vertebra), 2-finger width lateral to the lower edge.

Procedure: Insert the needle perpendicularly or obliquely into a depth of 0.5 to 1 cun, retaining it for 20 to 30 minutes.

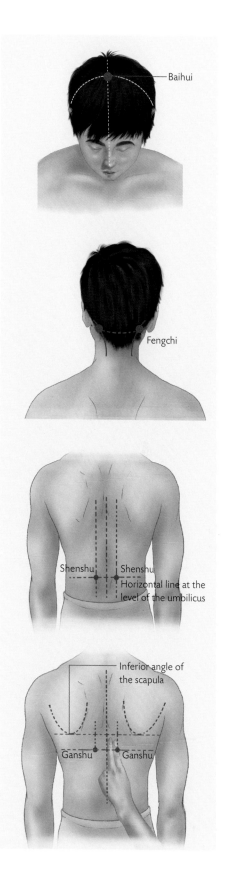

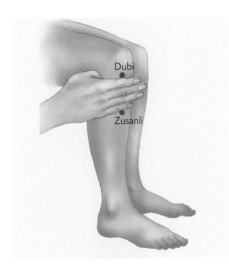

5. Zusanli Acupoint

Location: On the front lateral aspect of the lower leg, 3 cun (about 4-finger width) below the Dubi acupoint, 1-finger width lateral to the anterior crest of the tibia.

Quick location: Stand and bend over; use the tiger's mouth of hand on the same side to encircle the upper outer edge of the patella, with the remaining 4 fingers pointing downward, and the tip of the middle finger is this point.

Procedure: Insert the needle perpendicularly or obliquely into a depth of 0.5 to 1 cun, retaining it for 20 to 30 minutes.

Stomachache

Stomachache refers to the pain in the upper abdomen and epigastric region. The pathological focus of this condition is on the stomach, and the acupuncture treatment is centered on regulating the stomach and reliving pain. Patients with stomachaches should be mindful of their diet, avoiding spicy and irritating foods, and maintaining a positive emotional state.

The main acupuncture points for treating stomachache are Zhongwan, Zusanli, and Neiguan. Specific acupuncture points for different patterns are as follows:

Patterns	Diagnostic Features	Acupuncture Points
Excessive pathogen invading stomach	Sudden onset of stomach pain and bloating, with pain that worsens when pressed	Main acupoints + Weishu, Liangqiu
Spleen-stomach deficiency	Pain not prominent, but relieved when pressed	Main acupoints + Pishu, Guanyuan

Procedure: Conventional needle insertion.
Position: Supine position.

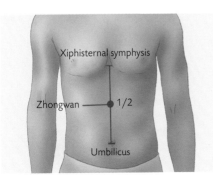

Main Acupoints

1. Zhongwan Acupoint

Location: In the upper abdomen, at the midpoint of the line connecting the xiphisternal symphysis with the umbilicus.

Procedure: Insert the needle perpendicularly into a depth of 0.5 to 1 cun, retaining it for 20 to 30 minutes.

2. Zusanli Acupoint

Location: On the front lateral aspect of the lower leg, 3 cun (about 4-finger width) below the Dubi acupoint, 1-finger width lateral to the anterior crest of the tibia.

Quick location: Stand and bend over; use the tiger's mouth of hand on the same side to encircle the upper outer edge of the patella, with the remaining 4 fingers pointing downward, and the tip of the middle finger is this point.

Procedure: Insert the needle perpendicularly into a depth of 1 to 2 cun, retaining it for 20 to 30 minutes.

3. Neiguan Acupoint

Location: On the palmar aspect of the forearm, along the line connecting the Quze acupoint and the Daling acupoint, 2 cun above the palmar wrist crease, between the palmaris longus tendon and the flexor carpi radialis tendon.

Quick location: 3-finger width above the palmar wrist crease, between the two major tendons.

Procedure: Insert the needle perpendicularly or obliquely into a depth of 0.5 to 1 cun, retaining it for 20 to 30 minutes.

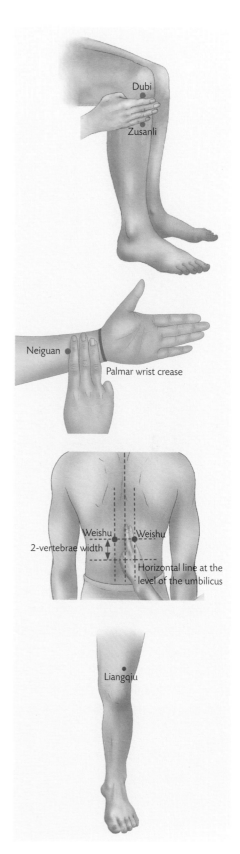

Excessive Pathogen Invading Stomach: Main Acupoints + Weishu, Liangqiu

1. Weishu Acupoint

Location: On the back, below the spinous process of the 12nd thoracic vertebra, 1.5 cun lateral to the posterior midline.

Quick location: 2 vertebrae above the intersection of the horizontal line at the level of the umbilicus and the spine, 2-finger width lateral to the lower edge.

Procedure: Insert the needle perpendicularly or obliquely into a depth of 0.5 to 1 cun, retaining it for 20 to 30 minutes.

2. Liangqiu Acupoint

Location: In the anterior thigh region, along the line connecting the anterior superior iliac spine and the lateral side of the basis patellae, 2 cun (3-finger width) above the basis patellae.

Quick location: Find the depression above the upper lateral edge of the patella when the lower limb is forcefully extended.

Procedure: Insert the needle perpendicularly into a depth of 1 to 1.2 cun, retaining it for 20 to 30 minutes.

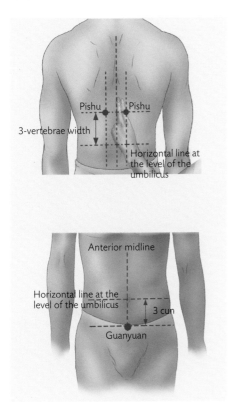

Spleen-Stomach Deficiency: Main Acupoints + Pishu, Guanyuan

1. Pishu Acupoint

Location: On the back, below the spinous process of the 11th thoracic vertebra, 1.5 cun lateral to the posterior midline.

Quick location: 3 vertebrae above the intersection of the horizontal line at the level of the umbilicus and the spine, 2-finger width lateral to the lower edge.

Procedure: Insert the needle perpendicularly or obliquely into a depth of 0.5 to 1 cun, retaining it for 20 to 30 minutes.

2. Guanyuan Acupoint

Location: In the lower abdomen, on the anterior midline, 3 cun (4-finger width) below the umbilicus.

Procedure: Insert the needle obliquely into a depth of 1.5 to 2 cun, retaining it for 20 to 30 minutes.

Emesis

Emesis is a condition characterized by upward counterflowing of stomach *qi* and the expulsion of stomach contents through the mouth. The pathological focus of this condition is on the stomach, and the acupuncture treatment is centered on regulating the stomach and alleviating vomiting symptoms. Patients are advised to focus on dietetic regulation in their daily routine, avoiding overeating as well as spicy, stimulating, cold, greasy, and sweet foods.

The main acupoints for addressing emesis are Zhongwan, Zusanli, and Neiguan. Specific acupuncture points for different patterns are as follows:

Patterns	Diagnostic Features	Acupuncture Points
Excessive pathogen invading stomach	Sudden onset, large amount of vomiting, and sour and foul-smelling vomitus	Main acupoints + Liangmen, Hegu
Spleen-stomach deficiency	Prolonged course of the disease, slow onset, small amount of vomiting, and less pronounced foul odor	Main acupoints + Pishu, Weishu

Procedure: Conventional needle insertion.

Position: Supine or lateral position.

Main Acupoints

1. Zhongwan Acupoint

Location: In the upper abdomen, at the midpoint of the line connecting the xiphisternal symphysis and the umbilicus.

Procedure: Insert the needle perpendicularly into a depth of 0.5 to 1 cun, retaining it for 20 to 30 minutes.

2. Zusanli Acupoint

Location: On the front lateral aspect of the lower leg, 3 cun (about 4-finger width) below the Dubi acupoint, 1-finger width lateral to the anterior crest of the tibia.

Quick location: Stand and bend over; use the tiger's mouth of hand on the same side to encircle the upper outer edge of the patella, with the remaining 4 fingers pointing downward, and the tip of the middle finger is this point.

Procedure: Insert the needle perpendicularly into a depth of 1.5 to 2 cun, retaining it for 20 to 30 minutes.

3. Neiguan Acupoint

Location: On the palmar aspect of the forearm, along the line connecting the Quze acupoint and the Daling acupoint, 2 cun above the palmar wrist crease, between the palmaris longus tendon and the flexor carpi radialis tendon.

Quick location: 3-finger width above the palmar wrist crease, between the two major tendons.

Procedure: Insert the needle perpendicularly into a depth of 0.5 to 1 cun, retaining it for 20 to 30 minutes.

Excessive Pathogen Invading Stomach:
Main Acupoints + Liangmen, Hegu

1. Liangmen Acupoint

Location: In the upper abdomen, 4 cun above the umbilicus, 2 cun lateral to the anterior midline (3-finger width).

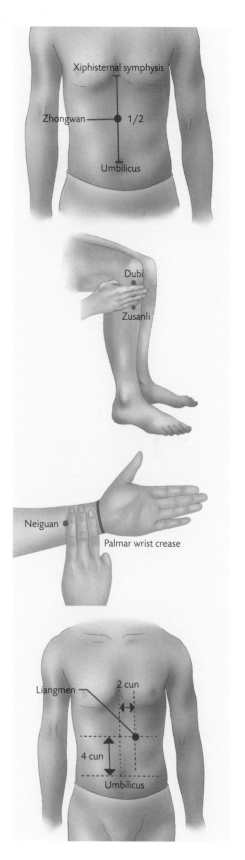

Quick location: While lying supine, locate the midpoint between the umbilicus and the xiphisternal symphysis (lower end of the sternum), then move horizontally to the side by 3-finger width.

Procedure: Insert the needle perpendicularly into a depth of 1 to 2.5 cun, retaining it for 20 to 30 minutes.

2. Hegu Acupoint

Location: On the dorsum of the hand, between the 1st and 2nd metacarpal bones, at the midpoint of the radial side on the 2nd metacarpal bone.

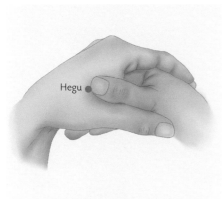

Quick location: Take the crease of the thumb interphalangeal joint of one hand and place it on the edge of the web between the thumb and forefinger of the other hand, where the tip of the thumb lands is Hegu acupoint.

Procedure: Insert the needle perpendicularly into a depth of 0.5 to 1 cun, retaining it for 20 to 30 minutes.

Spleen-Stomach Deficiency: Main Acupoints + Pishu, Weishu

1. Pishu Acupoint

Location: On the back, below the spinous process of the 11th thoracic vertebra, 1.5 cun lateral to the posterior midline.

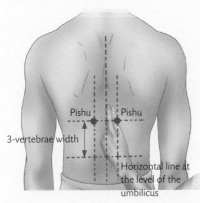

Quick location: 3 vertebrae above the intersection of the horizontal line at the level of the umbilicus and the spine, 2-finger width lateral to the lower edge.

Procedure: Insert the needle perpendicularly or obliquely into a depth of 0.5 to 1 cun, retaining it for 20 to 30 minutes.

2. Weishu Acupoint

Location: On the back, below the spinous process of the 12nd thoracic vertebra, 1.5 cun lateral to the posterior midline.

Quick location: 2 vertebrae above the intersection of the horizontal line at the level of the umbilicus and the spine, 2-finger width lateral to the lower edge.

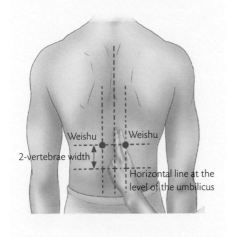

Procedure: Insert the needle perpendicularly or obliquely into a depth of 0.5 to 1 cun, retaining it for 20 to 30 minutes.

Hiccup

Hiccup, characterized by upward counterflowing of *qi*, continuous hiccup in the throat, short and frequent sound, and inability to control it, is a prominent clinical syndrome. The pathological focus of this condition is in the diaphragm, and the acupuncture treatment focuses on regulating *qi* and stomach functions, lowering adverse *qi* and halting hiccup. However, for cases of recurrent, chronic, and stubborn hiccup, it is essential to identify the underlying causes and implement tailored therapeutic interventions.

The main acupuncture points for treating hiccup are Zhongwan, Zusanli, Neiguan, Danzhong, Geshu, and Cuanzhu. Specific acupuncture points for different patterns are as follows:

Patterns	Diagnostic Features	Acupuncture Points
Excessive pathogen invading stomach	Strong hiccup sound	Main acupoints + Weishu, Neiting
Stomach-*yin* deficiency	Weak and intermittent hiccup sound	Main acupoints + Shenshu, Weishu

Procedure: Conventional needle insertion.
Position: Sitting position.

Main Acupoints

1. Zhongwan Acupoint

Location: In the upper abdomen, at the midpoint of the line connecting the xiphisternal symphysis and the umbilicus.

Procedure: Insert the needle perpendicularly or obliquely into a depth of 0.5 to 1 cun, retaining it for 20 to 30 minutes.

2. Zusanli Acupoint

Location: On the front lateral aspect of the lower leg, 3 cun (about 4-finger width) below the Dubi acupoint, 1-finger width lateral to the anterior crest of the tibia.

Quick location: Stand and bend over; use the tiger's mouth of hand on the same side to encircle the upper outer edge of the patella, with the remaining 4 fingers pointing downward, and the tip of the middle finger is this point.

Procedure: Insert the needle perpendicularly into a depth of 1 to 2 cun, retaining it for 20 to 30 minutes.

3. Neiguan Acupoint

Location: On the palmar aspect of the

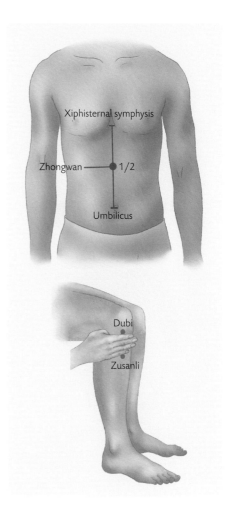

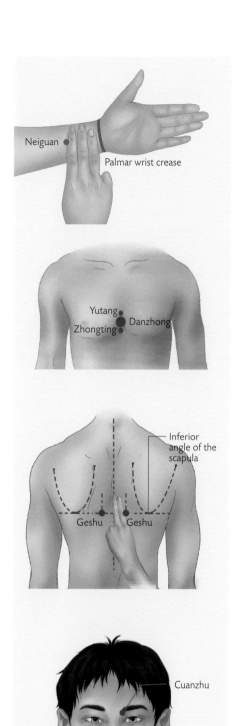

forearm, along the line connecting the Quze and the Daling acupoints, 2 cun above the palmar wrist crease, between the palmaris longus tendon and the flexor carpi radialis tendon.

Quick location: 3-finger width above the palmar wrist crease, between the two major tendons.

Procedure: Insert the needle perpendicularly or obliquely into a depth of 0.5 to 1 cun, retaining it for 20 to 30 minutes.

4. Danzhong Acupoint

Location: In the thorax, at the midpoint between the nipples, and horizontally at the 4th intercostal space.

Procedure: Employ skin-pinching up needle inserting method, and insert the needle horizontally into a depth of 0.3 to 0.5 cun, retaining it for 20 to 30 minutes.

5. Geshu Acupoint

Location: On the back, below the spinous process of the 7th thoracic vertebra, 1.5 cun lateral to the posterior midline.

Quick location: The intersection of the horizontal line drawn from the inferior angle of the scapula and the spine (the spinous process of the 7th thoracic vertebra), 2-finger width lateral to the lower edge.

Procedure: Insert the needle perpendicularly or obliquely into a depth of 0.5 to 1 cun, retaining it for 20 to 30 minutes.

6. Cuanzhu Acupoint

Location: In the depression at the inner tip of the eyebrows, at the supraorbital notch.

Procedure: Insert the needle horizontally or obliquely towards the middle of the eyebrow or the inner edge of the orbit, into a depth of 0.5 to 0.8 cun, retaining it for 20 to 30 minutes.

Excessive Pathogen Invading Stomach: Main Acupoints + Weishu, Neiting

1. Weishu Acupoint

Location: On the back, below the spinous

process of the 12nd thoracic vertebra, 1.5 cun lateral to the posterior midline.

Quick location: 2 vertebrae above the intersection of the horizontal line at the level of the umbilicus and the spine, 2-finger width lateral to the lower edge.

Procedure: Insert the needle perpendicularly or obliquely into a depth of 0.5 to 1 cun, retaining it for 20 to 30 minutes.

2. Neiting Acupoint

Location: On the dorsum of the foot, between the 2nd and 3rd toes, at the junction of the red and white flesh posterior to the toe web.

Procedure: Insert the needle perpendicularly or obliquely into a depth of 0.5 to 1 cun, retaining it for 20 to 30 minutes.

Stomach-*Yin* Deficiency: Main Acupoints + Pishu, Weishu

1. Pishu Acupoint

Location: On the back, below the spinous process of the 11th thoracic vertebra, 1.5 cun lateral to the posterior midline.

Quick location: 3 vertebrae above the intersection of the horizontal line at the level of the umbilicus and the spine, 2-finger width lateral to the lower edge.

Procedure: Insert the needle perpendicularly or obliquely into a depth of 0.5 to 1 cun, retaining it for 20 to 30 minutes.

2. Weishu Acupoint

Location: On the back, below the spinous process of the 12nd thoracic vertebra, 1.5 cun lateral to the posterior midline.

Quick location: 2 vertebrae above the intersection of the horizontal line at the level of the umbilicus and the spine, 2-finger width lateral to the lower edge.

Procedure: Insert the needle perpendicularly or obliquely into a depth of 0.5 to 1 cun, retaining it for 20 to 30 minutes.

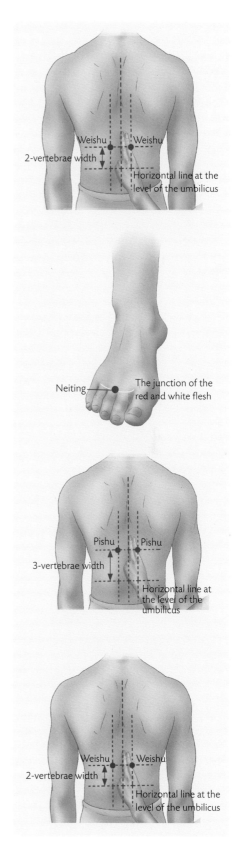

Diarrhea

Diarrhea is characterized by increased frequency of bowel movements and loose or undigested stools, sometimes even watery stools. The pathological focus of this condition is in the intestines and the main cause is dysfunction of spleen in transportation.

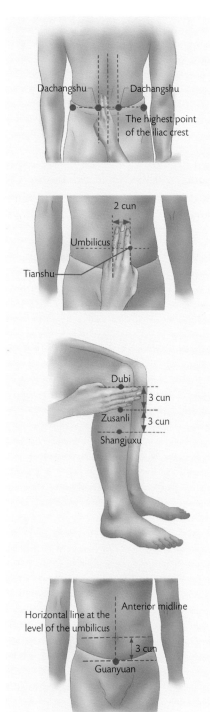

Acupuncture treatment focuses on strengthening the spleen, promoting fluid metabolism, regulating intestinal function, and alleviating diarrhea. During the treatment process, patients are advised to follow a bland diet, avoiding raw, cold, spicy, and stimulating foods.

Acupuncture points: Dachangshu, Tianshu, Shangjuxu, Guanyuan, and Shenque.

Procedure: Conventional needle insertion.

Position: Lateral position.

1. Dachangshu Acupoint

Location: At the waist, below the spinous process of the 4th lumbar vertebra, 1.5 cun lateral to the posterior midline.

Quick location: 2-finger width lateral to the intersection of the spine and the line connecting the highest point of the iliac crest on both sides.

Procedure: Insert the needle perpendicularly or obliquely into a depth of 0.5 to 1 cun, retaining it for 20 to 30 minutes.

2. Tianshu Acupoint

Location: In the abdomen, 2 cun (3-finger width) lateral to the umbilicus.

Procedure: Insert the needle perpendicularly or obliquely into a depth of 0.5 to 1 cun, retaining it for 20 to 30 minutes.

3. Shangjuxu Acupoint

Location: On the front lateral aspect of the lower leg, 6 cun (about two 4-finger width) below the Dubi acupoint, 1-finger width lateral to the anterior tibia.

Procedure: Insert the needle perpendicularly or obliquely into a depth of 0.5 to 1 cun, retaining it for 20 to 30 minutes.

4. Guanyuan Acupoint

Location: In the lower abdomen, on the anterior midline, 3 cun (4-finger width) below the umbilicus.

Procedure: Employ the heavy moxibustion with large moxa cones, wherein moxa cones are consecutively applied for approximately 6 hours, repeated for 3 consecutive days.

5. Shenque Acupoint

Location: In the center of the umbilicus.

Procedure: Employ the heavy moxibustion with large moxa cones.

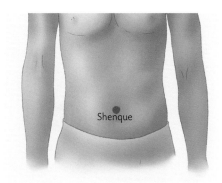

Constipation

Constipation refers to the condition characterized by dry and difficult-to-pass stool, with either a prolonged bowel movement cycle or delayed time, or difficulty in defecation despite the urge to do so. The pathological focus of this condition is in the large intestine, and the acupuncture treatment focuses on regulating intestinal function and promoting bowel movements.

The main acupuncture points for treating constipation are Tianshu, Dachangshu, Shangjuxu, Zhigou, Zhaohai, and Baliao. Specific acupuncture points for different patterns are as follows:

Patterns	Diagnostic Features	Acupuncture Points
Excessive constipation	Dry stool, difficult to pass	Main acupoints + Hegu, Zhongwan
Deficient constipation	Despite the urge to defecate, the bowel movement is not smooth and the stool is not dry or hard	Main acupoints + Guanyuan, Pishu

Procedure: Conventional needle insertion.

Position: Lateral position.

Main Acupoints

1. Tianshu Acupoint

Location: In the abdomen, 2 cun (3-finger width) lateral to the umbilicus.

Procedure: Insert the needle perpendicularly into a depth of 1 to 1.5 cun, retaining it for 20 to 30 minutes.

2. Dachangshu Acupoint

Location: At the waist, below the spinous process of the 4th lumbar vertebra, 1.5 cun lateral to the posterior midline.

Quick location: 2-finger width lateral to the

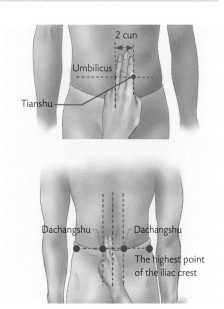

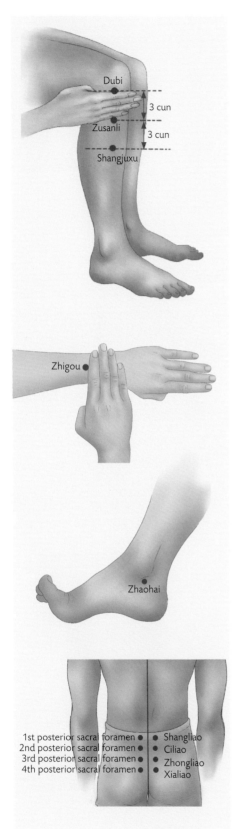

intersection of the spine and the line connecting the highest point of the iliac crest on both sides.

Procedure: Insert the needle perpendicularly or obliquely into a depth of 0.5 to 1 cun, retaining it for 20 to 30 minutes.

3. Shangjuxu Acupoint

Location: On the front lateral aspect of the lower leg, 6 cun (about two 4-finger width) below the Dubi acupoint, 1-finger width lateral to the anterior tibia.

Procedure: Insert the needle perpendicularly or obliquely into a depth of 0.5 to 1 cun, retaining it for 20 to 30 minutes.

4. Zhigou Acupoint

Location: On the back of the arm, along the line connecting the Yangchi point (see page 99) and the elbow tip, 3 cun (4-finger width) on the dorsal wrist crease, between the ulna and the radius.

Procedure: Insert the needle perpendicularly or obliquely into a depth of 0.5 to 1 cun, retaining it for 20 to 30 minutes.

5. Zhaohai Acupoint

Location: On the medial aspect of the foot, 1 cun below the prominence of the medial malleolus in the depression.

Procedure: Insert the needle perpendicularly or obliquely into a depth of 0.5 to 1 cun, retaining it for 20 to 30 minutes.

6. Baliao Acupoints

Location: These acupuncture points are collectively referred to as Shangliao, Ciliao, Zhongliao, and Xialiao, totaling eight points distributed bilaterally within the first to fourth posterior sacral foramina.

Procedure: Insert the needle perpendicularly into a depth of 1 to 1.5 cun, retaining it for 20 to 30 minutes.

Excessive Constipation: Main Acupoints + Hegu, Zhongwan

1. Hegu Acupoint

Location: On the dorsum of the hand, between

the 1st and 2nd metacarpal bones, at the midpoint of the radial side on the 2nd metacarpal bone.

Quick location: Take the crease of the thumb interphalangeal joint of one hand and place it on the edge of the web between the thumb and forefinger of the other hand, where the tip of the thumb lands is Hegu acupoint.

Procedure: Insert the needle perpendicularly or obliquely into a depth of 0.5 to 1 cun, retaining it for 20 to 30 minutes.

2. Zhongwan Acupoint

Location: In the upper abdomen, at the midpoint between the xiphisternal symphysis and the umbilicus.

Procedure: Insert the needle perpendicularly or obliquely into a depth of 0.5 to 1 cun, retaining it for 20 to 30 minutes.

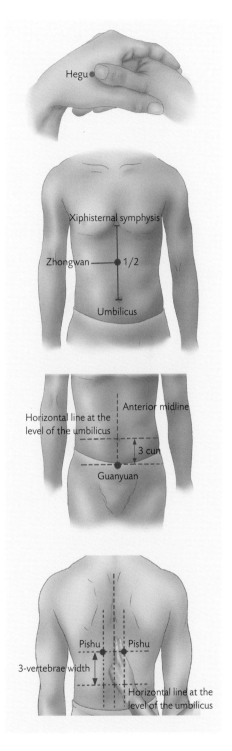

Deficient Constipation: Main Acupoints + Guanyuan, Pishu

1. Guanyuan Acupoint

Location: In the lower abdomen, on the anterior midline, 3 cun (4-finger width) below the umbilicus.

Procedure: Insert the needle perpendicularly or obliquely into a depth of 1 to 1.5 cun, retaining it for 20 to 30 minutes.

2. Pishu Acupoint

Location: On the back, below the spinous process of the 11th thoracic vertebra, 1.5 cun lateral to the posterior midline.

Quick location: 3 vertebrae above the intersection of the horizontal line at the level of the umbilicus and the spine, 2-finger width lateral to the lower edge.

Procedure: Insert the needle perpendicularly or obliquely into a depth of 0.5 to 1 cun, retaining it for 20 to 30 minutes.

 Physician's advice: ① Develop a routine of regular bowel movements. ② Incorporate a variety of vegetables, fruits, and particularly foods rich in dietary fiber into your daily diet.

Insomnia

Insomnia is characterized by the consistent inability to achieve normal sleep patterns. Mild cases struggle with falling asleep, easily waking up during the night, and finding it difficult to return to sleep. Severe cases experience prolonged periods of sleeplessness throughout the night. The pathological focus of this condition is in the heart, and the acupuncture treatment focuses on harmonizing *yin* and *yang*, calming the mind and soothing the spirit.

The main acupuncture points for treating insomnia are Baihui, Shenmen, Sanyinjiao, Anmian, and Sishencong. Specific acupuncture points for different patterns are as follows:

Patterns	Diagnostic Features	Acupuncture Points
Disturbance of phlegm-fire	Concurrent manifestations of irritability, restlessness, headache, dizziness, bitter taste with excessive phlegm, red tongue with yellow coating	Main acupoints + Taichong, Fenglong
Heart-kidney disharmony	Concurrent manifestations of feverishness in palms and soles, dizziness, tinnitus, soreness and weakness in the waist and knees, red tongue with little coating	Main acupoints + Xinshu, Shenshu
Deficiency of both heart and spleen	Concurrent manifestations of palpitations, forgetfulness, dizziness, blurred vision, fatigue, dull complexion, loss of appetite, loose stools, pale tongue with white coating	Main acupoints + Xinshu, Geshu

Procedure: Conventional needle insertion.
Position: Supine position.

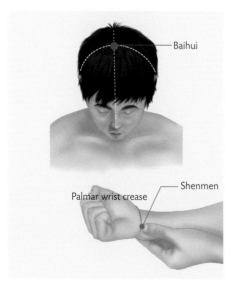

Baihui

Shenmen

Palmar wrist crease

Main Acupoints

1. Baihui Acupoint

Location: On the head, at the intersection of the line connecting both ear tips and the midline of the head.

Procedure: Insert the needle horizontally into a depth of 0.5 to 0.8 cun, retaining it for 20 to 30 minutes.

2. Shenmen Acupoint

Location: On the ulnar side (little finger side) along the palmar wrist crease, in the depression of the radial side (thumb side) of the flexor carpi radialis tendon.

Procedure: Insert the needle

perpendicularly or obliquely into a depth of 0.5 to 1 cun, retaining it for 20 to 30 minutes.

3. Sanyinjiao Acupoint

Location: On the medial aspect of the lower leg, 3 cun (4-finger width) above the prominence of the medial malleolus, posterior to the medial border of the tibia.

Procedure: Insert the needle perpendicularly or obliquely into a depth of 0.5 to 1 cun; retain the needle for 20 to 30 minutes.

4. Anmian Acupoint

Location: The midpoint along the line connecting the Yifeng acupoint and the Fengchi acupoint.

Procedure: Insert the needle perpendicularly into a depth of 0.8 to 1.2 cun, retaining it for 20 to 30 minutes.

5. Sishencong Acupoints

Location: On the top of the head, 1 cun (1-finger width) in front, behind, to the left, and to the right of the Baihui acupoint, totaling four acupuncture points.

Procedure: Inserted the needle horizontally towards the Baihui acupoint or in the surrounding direction, into a depth of 0.5 to 0.8 cun, retaining it for 20 to 30 minutes.

Disturbance of Phlegm-Fire: Main Acupoints + Taichong, Fenglong

1. Taichong Acupoint

Location: On the dorsum of the foot, in the depression in front of the junction between the 1st and 2nd metatarsal bones.

Quick location: On the dorsum of the foot, push upward along the crease between the 1st and 2nd toes. The depression felt is the Taichong acupoint.

Procedure: Insert the needle perpendicularly into a depth of 0.5 to 0.8 cun, retaining it for 20 to 30 minutes.

2. Fenglong Acupoint

Location: On the front lateral aspect of

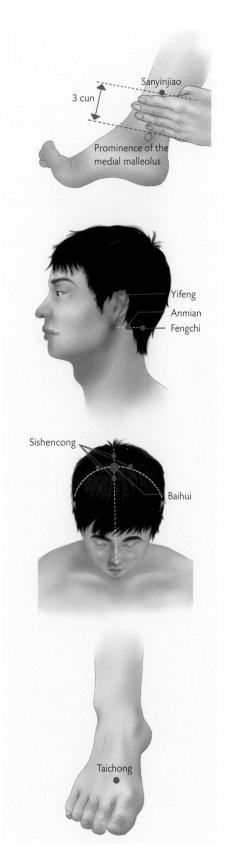

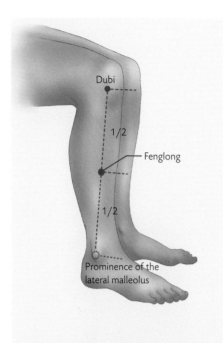

Dubi

1/2

Fenglong

1/2

Prominence of the lateral malleolus

the lower leg, 8 cun above the prominence of the lateral malleolus, 2-finger width from the anterior edge of the tibia.

Quick location: Bend the knee, draw a line between Dubi acupoint and the prominence of the lateral malleolus, and find the midpoint of the line.

Procedure: Insert the needle perpendicularly or obliquely into a depth of 0.5 to 1 cun, retaining it for 20 to 30 minutes.

Heart-Kidney Disharmony: Main Acupoints + Xinshu, Shenshu

1. Xinshu Acupoint

Location: On the back, below the spinous process of the 5th thoracic vertebra, 1.5 cun lateral to the posterior midline.

Quick location: 2 vertebrae above the intersection of the horizontal line drawn from the inferior angle of the scapula and the spine (the spinous process of the 7th thoracic vertebra), 2-finger width lateral to the lower edge.

Procedure: Insert the needle obliquely into a depth of 0.5 to 0.8 cun, avoiding deep insertion to prevent injury to vital internal organs. Retain the needle for 20 to 30 minutes.

2. Shenshu Acupoint

Location: In the lumbar region, below the spinous process of the 2nd lumbar vertebra, 1.5 cun lateral to the posterior midline.

Quick location: 2-finger width lateral to the intersection of the horizontal line at the level of the umbilicus and the spine.

Procedure: Insert the needle perpendicularly into a depth of 0.5 to 1 cun, retaining it for 20 to 30 minutes.

Deficiency of Both Heart and Spleen: Main Acupoints + Xinshu, Geshu

1. Xinshu Acupoint

Location: On the back, below the spinous

The highest point of the junction between the back of the neck and the upper back

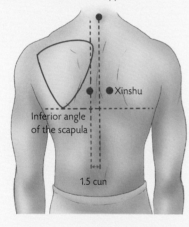

Xinshu

Inferior angle of the scapula

1.5 cun

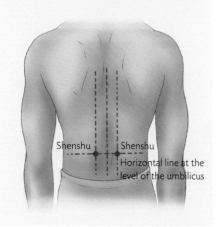

Shenshu

Shenshu

Horizontal line at the level of the umbilicus

process of the 5th thoracic vertebra, 1.5 cun lateral to the posterior midline.

Quick location: 2 vertebrae above the intersection of the horizontal line drawn from the inferior angle of the scapula and the spine (the spinous process of the 7th thoracic vertebra), 2-finger width lateral to the lower edge.

Procedure: Insert the needle obliquely into a depth of 0.5 to 0.8 cun, avoiding deep insertion to prevent injury to internal vital organs. Retain the needle for 20 to 30 minutes.

2. Geshu Acupoint

Location: On the back, below the spinous process of the 7th thoracic vertebra, 1.5 cun lateral to the posterior midline.

Quick location: The intersection of the horizontal line drawn from the inferior angle of the scapula and the spine (the spinous process of the 7th thoracic vertebra), 2-finger width lateral to the lower edge.

Procedure: Insert the needle perpendicularly into a depth of 0.5 to 1 cun, retaining it for 20 to 30 minutes.

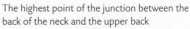
The highest point of the junction between the back of the neck and the upper back

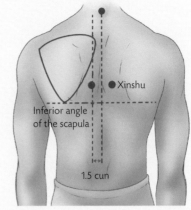
Inferior angle of the scapula · Xinshu · 1.5 cun

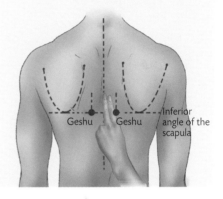
Geshu · Geshu · Inferior angle of the scapula

Physician's advice: ① Before treatment, identify the underlying cause of the ailment and pursue a scientifically sound course of treatment. ② Encourage patients to establish consistent and structured daily routines. ③ Avoid eating stimulating foods and engaging in vigorous exercise before bedtime.

Headache

Headache is a type of ailment characterized by self-perceived pain in the head. The pathology focus of this condition is in the head, as the three *yang* meridians of hand and foot, the Jueyin Liver Meridian of Foot, and the Governor Vessel all course through this region. Therefore, these meridians are intricately linked to headaches. Acupuncture treatment focuses on harmonizing *qi* and blood, promoting meridian circulation and alleviating pain.

Specific acupuncture points for different patterns are as follows:

Patterns	Diagnostic Features	Acupuncture Points
Yangming headache	Pain localized in the forehead, brow ridge, and root of the nose	Touwei, Yintang, Yangbai, Hegu, Ashi acupoints
Shaoyang headache	Pain localized on the side of the head	Taiyang, Sizhukong, Fengchi, Waiguan, Ashi acupoints
Taiyang headache	Pain localized at the back of the head or extending down to the neck	Tianzhu, Houding, Fengchi, Houxi, Ashi acupoints
Jueyin headache	Pain localized at the top of the head or extending to the eye connector	Baihui, Sishencong, Taichong, Ashi acupoints

Procedure: Conventional needle insertion. Pay attention to the angle and depth of needle insertion for Tianzhu, Fengchi, and other neck and nape acupuncture points.

Position: Lateral position.

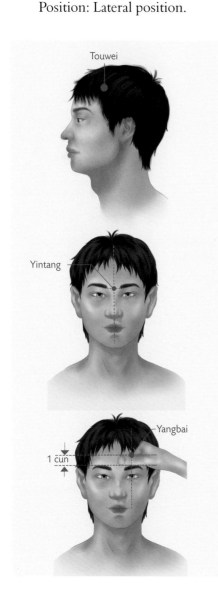

Yangming Headache

1. Touwei Acupoint

Location: On the lateral aspect of the head, 0.5 cun above the hairline at the temple, 4.5 cun lateral to the midline of the head.

Procedure: Insert the needle horizontally into a depth of 0.5 to 1 cun, retaining it for 20 to 30 minutes.

2. Yintang Acupoint

Location: On the forehead, at the midpoint between the eyebrows.

Procedure: Utilize the skin-pinching up needle inserting method to gently pinch up the local skin, and insert the needle horizontally and downward into a depth of 0.3 to 0.5 cun, retaining it for 20 to 30 minutes.

3. Yangbai Acupoint

Location: On the forehead, directly above the pupil, 1 cun (1-finger width) above the eyebrow.

Procedure: Utilize the skin-pinching up needle inserting method, and insert the needle horizontally towards the pupil direction into a depth of 0.5 to 0.8 cun, retaining it for 20 to 30 minutes.

4. Hegu Acupoint

Location: On the dorsum of the hand, between the 1st and 2nd metacarpal bones, at the midpoint of the radial side on the 2nd metacarpal bone.

Quick location: Take the crease of the thumb interphalangeal joint of one hand and place it on the edge of the web between the thumb and forefinger of the other hand, where the tip of the thumb lands is Hegu acupoint.

Procedure: Insert the needle perpendicularly or obliquely into a depth of 0.5 to 1 cun, retaining it for 20 to 30 minutes.

5. Ashi Acupoint

Location: The tender point serves as the acupuncture point, meaning the needle is inserted directly at the site of pain.

Procedure: Insert the needle perpendicularly or obliquely into a depth of 0.5 to 1 cun, retaining it for 20 to 30 minutes.

Shaoyang Headache

1. Taiyang Acupoint

Location: In the temporal region of the head, between the tip of the eyebrow and the outer canthus, in the depression approximately 1-finger width backwards.

Procedure: Insert the needle perpendicularly into a depth of 0.3 to 0.5 cun, retaining it for 20 to 30 minutes.

2. Sizhukong Acupoint

Location: Situated in the depression at the tip of the eyebrow.

Procedure: Insert the needle horizontally towards the Shuaigu acupoint into a depth of 1 to 2 cun, retaining it for 20 to 30 minutes. (Shuaigu acupoint is located 1.5 cun above the apex of the ear, extending towards the hairline.)

3. Fengchi Acupoint

Location: In the posterior neck region, below the occipital bone, in the depression between the upper end of the sternocleidomastoid muscle and the trapezius muscle.

Quick location: Sit upright, and the

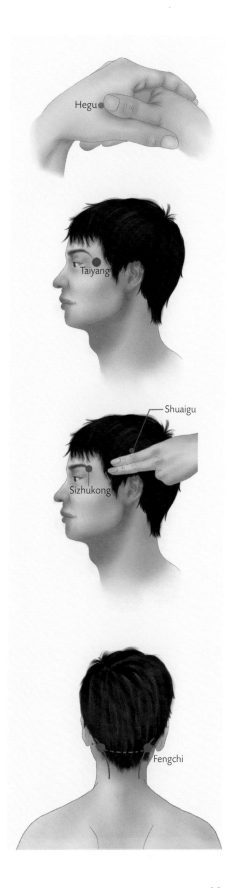

acupoint is situated in the depression on the lateral edge of the two major tendons below the occipital bone, level with the earlobe.

Procedure: Insert the needle obliquely towards the tip of the nose with the tip of the needle slightly downward, into a depth of 0.5 to 0.8 cun, or insert the needle horizontally towards the Fengfu acupoint (see page 133), retaining it for 20 to 30 minutes.

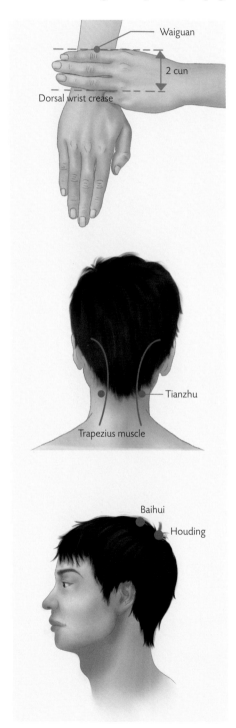

4. Waiguan Acupoint

Location: On the dorsum of the forearm, along the line connecting the Yangchi point (see page 99) and the elbow tip, 2 cun (3-finger width) above the dorsal wrist crease, between the ulna and radius (two major bones).

Procedure: Insert the needle perpendicularly or obliquely into a depth of 0.5 to 1 cun, retaining it for 20 to 30 minutes.

5. Ashi Acupoint

Location: The tender point serves as the acupuncture point, meaning the needle is inserted directly at the site of pain.

Procedure: Insert the needle perpendicularly or obliquely into a depth of 0.5 to 1 cun, retaining it for 20 to 30 minutes.

Taiyang Headache

1. Tianzhu Acupoint

Location: On the nape, in the depression of the posterior hairline lateral to the trapezius muscle, approximately 1.3 cun lateral to the midline of the posterior hairline.

Quick location: Sit upright with the head lowered. Palpate the outer edge of the two major tendons on the posterior neck. The depression at the edge of the posterior hairline marks the location of this acupoint.

Procedure: Insert the needle perpendicularly or obliquely into a depth of 0.5 to 0.8 cun. Avoid inward and upward needle insertion to prevent injury to the medulla oblongata. Retain the needle for 20 to 30 minutes.

2. Houding Acupoint

Location: 5.5 cun directly above the midline of the posterior hairline.

Quick location: 2-finger width behind the Baihui acupoint, on the midline.

Procedure: Insert the needle horizontally into a depth of 0.5 to 0.8 cun, retaining it for 20 to 30 minutes.

3. Fengchi Acupoint

Location: In the posterior neck region, below the occipital bone, in the depression between the upper end of the sternocleidomastoid muscle and the trapezius muscle.

Quick location: Sit upright, and the acupoint is situated in the depression on the lateral edge of the two major tendons below the occipital bone, level with the earlobe.

Procedure: Insert the needle obliquely towards the tip of the nose with the tip of the needle slightly downward, into a depth of 0.5 to 0.8 cun, or insert the needle horizontally towards the Fengfu point (see page 133), retaining it for 20 to 30 minutes.

4. Houxi Acupoint

Location: On the ulnar side of the palm, with a slight fist, at the posterior margin of the 5th metacarpophalangeal joint, at the junction of the red and white flesh on the ulnar side of the palmar crease.

Procedure: Insert the needle perpendicularly or obliquely into a depth of 0.5 to 1 cun, retaining it for 20 to 30 minutes.

5. Ashi Acupoint

Location: The tender point serves as the acupuncture point, meaning the needle is inserted directly at the site of pain.

Procedure: Insert the needle perpendicularly or obliquely into a depth of 0.5 to 1 cun, retaining it for 20 to 30 minutes.

Jueyin Headache

1. Baihui Acupoint

Location: On the head, at the intersection of the line connecting both ear tips and the midline of the head.

Procedure: Insert the needle horizontally into a depth of 0.5 to 0.8 cun, retaining it for 20 to 30 minutes.

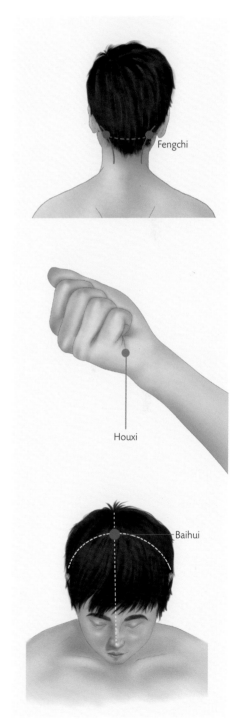

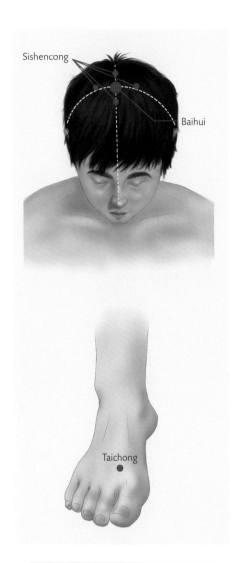

Sishencong

Baihui

Taichong

2. Sishencong Acupoints

Location: On the top of the head, 1 cun (1-finger width) in front, behind, to the left, and to the right of the Baihui acupoint, totaling four acupuncture points.

Procedure: Inserted the needle horizontally towards the Baihui acupoint or in the surrounding direction, into a depth of 0.5 to 0.8 cun, retaining it for 20 to 30 minutes.

3. Taichong Acupoint

Location: On the dorsum of the foot, in the depression in front of the junction between the 1st and 2nd metatarsal bones.

Quick location: On the dorsum of the foot, push upward along the crease between the 1st and 2nd toes. The depression felt is the Taichong acupoint.

Procedure: Insert the needle perpendicularly or obliquely into a depth of 0.5 to 1 cun, retaining it for 20 to 30 minutes.

4. Ashi Acupoint

Location: The tender point serves as the acupuncture point, meaning the needle is inserted directly at the site of pain.

Procedure: Insert the needle perpendicularly or obliquely into a depth of 0.5 to 1 cun, retaining it for 20 to 30 minutes.

 Physician's advice: ① Acupuncture shows promising results in treating functional headaches (often lacking clear causes, caused by disorders of brain neural regulation and vascular dysfunction), migraines, herpes zoster neuralgia, premenstrual and menstrual headaches. ② Before treatment, identify the underlying cause and opt for tailored therapeutic approaches. ③ During the treatment period, it's advised to abstain from smoking and alcohol consumption while engaging in appropriate physical exercise.

Spermatorrhea

Spermatorrhea refers to the frequent discharge of semen without sexual intercourse. Wet dreams are referred to as "nocturnal emission," while semen discharge during wakefulness is termed "night emission." For unmarried or married adult males who do not engage in regular sexual activity, experiencing 1 to 2 episodes of spermatorrhea per month is considered normal, but if it occurs more than twice a week, treatment is necessary. The pathology focus of this condition is in the kidneys, and acupuncture treatment focuses on regulating kidney function and preserving essence.

The main acupuncture points for treating spermatorrhea are Zhongji, Shenshu, Taixi, and Sanyinjiao. Specific acupuncture points for different patterns are as follows:

Patterns	Diagnostic Features	Acupuncture Points
Insufficiency of heart and kidney	Frequent spermatorrhea, pale complexion, palpitations, forgetfulness, insomnia, soreness and weakness of the waist and knees, pale tongue with thin coating	Main acupoints + Fuliu, Xinshu
Hyperactivity of fire due to *yin* deficiency	Frequent nocturnal emission, restlessness and heat in the heart, poor sleep quality, red tongue with little coating	Main acupoints + Shenmen, Ran'gu
Dampness-heat diffusing downward	Frequent nocturnal emission, semen leakage after urination, bitter taste in the mouth and desire to drink water, discomfort in the lower abdomen, red tongue with yellow and greasy coating	Main acupoints + Yinlingquan

Procedure: Conventional needle insertion.
Position: Supine position.

Main Acupoints

1. Zhongji Acupoint

Location: In the lower abdomen, on the anterior midline, 4 cun below the umbilicus.

Quick location: 1-finger width below Guanyuan acupoint.

Procedure: Insert the needle perpendicularly into a depth of 1 to 1.5 cun, retaining it for 20 to 30 minutes.

2. Shenshu Acupoint

Location: In the lumbar region, below the spinous process of the 2nd lumbar vertebra, 1.5 cun lateral to the posterior midline.

Quick location: 2-finger width lateral to the intersection of the horizontal line at the level of the umbilicus and the spine.

Procedure: Insert the needle perpendicularly or obliquely into a depth of 0.5 to 1 cun, retaining it for 20 to 30 minutes.

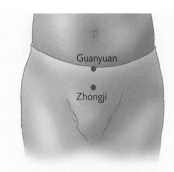

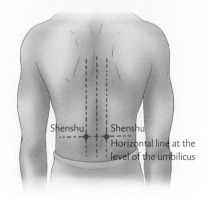

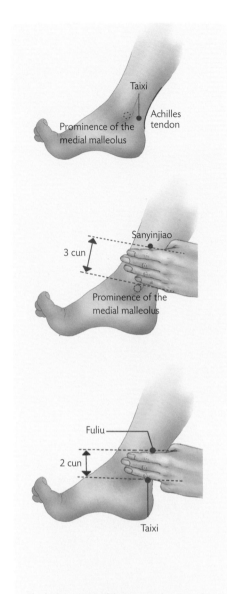

3. Taixi Acupoint

Location: On the medial aspect of the foot, in the depression between the prominence of the lateral malleolus and the Achilles tendon.

Procedure: Insert the needle perpendicularly or obliquely into a depth of 0.5 to 1 cun, retaining it for 20 to 30 minutes.

4. Sanyinjiao Acupoint

Location: On the medial aspect of the lower leg, 3 cun (4-finger width) above the prominence of the medial malleolus, posterior to the medial border of the tibia.

Procedure: Insert the needle perpendicularly or obliquely into a depth of 0.5 to 1 cun; retain the needle for 20 to 30 minutes.

Insufficiency of Heart and Kidney: Main Acupoints + Fuliu, Xinshu

1. Fuliu Acupoint

Location: On the medial aspect of the lower leg, 2 cun directly above the Taixi acupoint, in front of the Achilles tendon.

Quick location: About 2 cun (3-finger width) above the midpoint between the prominence of the medial malleolus and the posterior edge of the Achilles tendon (Taixi acupoint).

Procedure: Insert the needle perpendicularly or obliquely into a depth of 0.5 to 1 cun, retaining it for 20 to 30 minutes.

2. Xinshu Acupoint

Location: On the back, below the spinous process of the 5th thoracic vertebra, 1.5 cun lateral to the posterior midline.

Quick location: 2 vertebrae above the intersection of the horizontal line drawn from the inferior angle of the scapula and the spine (the spinous process of the 7th thoracic vertebra), 2-finger width lateral to the lower edge.

Procedure: Insert the needle obliquely into a depth of 0.5 to 0.8 cun, avoiding deep insertion to prevent injury to vital internal organs. Retain the needle for 20 to 30 minutes.

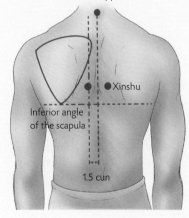

Hyperactivity of Fire Due to *Yin* Deficiency: Main Acupoints + Shenmen, Ran'gu

1. Shenmen Acupoint

Location: On the ulnar side (little finger side) along the palmar wrist crease, in the depression of the radial side (thumb side) of the flexor carpi radialis tendon.

Procedure: Insert the needle perpendicularly or obliquely into a depth of 0.5 to 1 cun, retaining it for 20 to 30 minutes.

2. Ran'gu Acupoint

Location: On the medial edge of the foot, at the junction of the red and white flesh below the tuberosity of the navicular bone.

Quick location: Find the prominent bony mark known as the navicular bone on the anterior and inferior aspect of the medial malleolus, and the acupoint is located in the depression anterior and inferior to the bone.

Procedure: Insert the needle obliquely into a depth of 0.5 to 0.8 cun, retaining it for 20 to 30 minutes.

Dampness-Heat Diffusing Downward: Main Acupoints + Yinlingquan

Yinlingquan Acupoint

Location: On the medial aspect of the lower leg, in the depression below the posterior aspect of the medial malleolus of the tibia.

Quick location: Use the index finger to move upward along the medial aspect of the lower leg, reaching the depression where the tibia bends inward and upward, just below the knee joint.

Procedure: Insert the needle perpendicularly or obliquely into a depth of 1.5 to 2 cun, retaining it for 20 to 30 minutes.

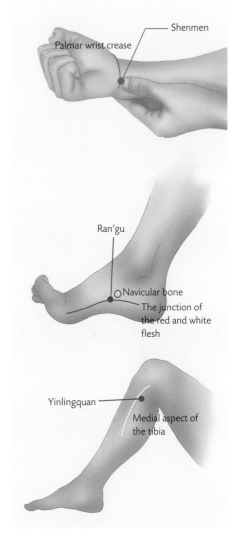

 Physician's advice: ① While treating functional spermatorrhea, it's essential to address the patient's mental burden; for organic diseases, treating the underlying condition is crucial. ② Simultaneously with treatment, abstaining from masturbation is advised.

CHAPTER FIVE

Acupuncture Treatment for Orthopedic Conditions

This chapter covers common chronic bone injuries such as cervical spondylosis, stiff neck, shoulder periarthritis, as well as acute emergencies such as lumbar sprain and joint sprain. Please note that acupuncture should be performed by professionals. Please exercise caution, ensuring that the intensity of acupuncture is within the patient's comfort level.

Cervical Spondylosis

Cervical spondylosis, characterized by changes such as cervical osteophyte formation, calcification of cervical ligaments, and degeneration of cervical intervertebral discs, results in a syndrome of symptoms and signs caused by the stimulation or compression of cervical nerves, spinal cord, and blood vessels. This condition progresses slowly and manifests primarily as pain in the head, neck, shoulder, back, and upper limbs, as well as progressive sensory and motor disorders in the limbs.

The pathological focus of this condition is in the neck muscles and bones, and acupuncture treatment focuses on relieving the rigidity of muscles and activating collaterals.

The main acupoints are Jiaji, Tianzhu, and Houxi. Specific acupuncture points for different patterns are as follows:

Patterns	Diagnostic Features	Acupuncture Points
Blockade caused by wind-cold	Prolonged exposure to damp environments or sleeping with exposed shoulders in cold conditions, resulting in soreness and pain in the shoulders and arms, aggravated by cold; pale tongue with white coating	Main acupoints + Fengmen, Dazhui
Blood vessel stasis and obstruction	Typically seen after external trauma, presenting as neck stiffness, shoulder and arm pain, with tenderness in the upper and lower scapular fossa and shoulder peak; dark purplish tongue with petechiae	Main acupoints + Geshu, Hegu
Liver-kidney deficiency	Symptoms worsen after fatigue, with soreness and weakness in the waist and knees, dizziness and tinnitus; red tongue with little coating	Main acupoints + Ganshu, Shenshu

Procedure: Even reinforcing-reducing method.

Position: Prone position.

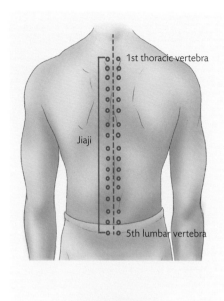

1st thoracic vertebra

Jiaji

5th lumbar vertebra

Main Acupoints

1. Jiaji Acupoint

Location: Below the spinous process of the 1st thoracic vertebra to the 5th lumbar vertebra, 0.5 cun (half-finger width) lateral to the posterior midline.

Procedure: Insert the needle perpendicularly or obliquely into a depth of 0.5 to 0.8 cun. Avoid inward and upward needle insertion to prevent injury to the medulla oblongata. Retain the needle for 20 to 30 minutes.

2. Tianzhu Acupoint

Location: On the nape, in the depression of the posterior hairline lateral to the trapezius muscle, approximately 1.3 cun lateral to the midline of the posterior hairline.

Quick location: Sit upright with the head lowered. Palpate the outer edge of the two major tendons on the posterior neck. The depression at the edge of the posterior hairline marks the location of this acupuncture point.

Procedure: Insert the needle perpendicularly or obliquely into a depth of 0.5 to 0.8 cun. Avoid inward and upward needle insertion to prevent injury to the medulla oblongata. Retain the needle for 20 to 30 minutes.

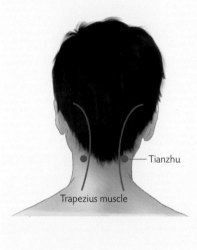

Tianzhu

Trapezius muscle

3. Houxi Acupoint

Location: On the ulnar side of the palm, with a slight fist, at the posterior margin of the 5th metacarpophalangeal joint, at the junction of the red and white flesh on the ulnar side of the palmar crease.

Procedure: Insert the needle perpendicularly or obliquely into a depth of 0.5 to 1 cun, retaining it for 20 to 30 minutes.

Blockade Caused by Wind-Cold: Main Acupoints + Fengmen, Dazhui

1. Fengmen Acupoint

Location: On the back, below the spinous

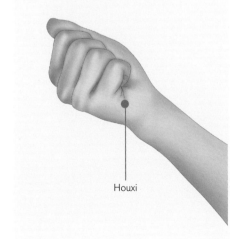

Houxi

process of the 2nd thoracic vertebra, 1.5 cun lateral to the posterior midline.

Quick location: Lower the head, and the highest point of the junction between the back of the neck and the upper back corresponds to the spinous process of the 7th cervical vertebra. Count down 2 vertebrae, the acupoint is situated 2-finger width beside the lower edge.

Procedure: Insert the needle obliquely into a depth of 0.5 to 0.8 cun, retaining it for 20 to 30 minutes.

2. Dazhui Acupoint

Location: In the spinal area, below the spinous process of the 7th cervical vertebra, on the posterior midline.

Quick location: Lower the head, and the highest point of the junction between the back of the neck and the upper back corresponds to the spinous process of the 7th cervical vertebra, and the depression below it is the Dazhui acupoint.

Procedure: Insert the needle perpendicularly or obliquely into a depth of 0.5 to 1 cun, retaining it for 20 to 30 minutes.

Blood Vessels Stasis and Obstruction: Main Acupoints + Geshu, Hegu

1. Geshu Acupoint

Location: On the back, below the spinous process of the 7th thoracic vertebra, 1.5 cun lateral to the posterior midline.

Quick location: The intersection of the horizontal line drawn from the inferior angle of the scapula and the spine (the spinous process of the 7th thoracic vertebra), 2-finger width lateral to the lower edge.

Procedure: Insert the needle perpendicularly into a depth of 0.5 to 1 cun, retaining it for 20 to 30 minutes.

2. Hegu Acupoint

Location: On the dorsum of the hand,

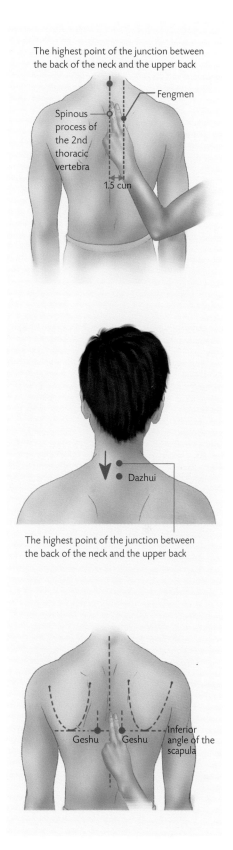

The highest point of the junction between the back of the neck and the upper back

Fengmen

Spinous process of the 2nd thoracic vertebra

1.5 cun

The highest point of the junction between the back of the neck and the upper back

Dazhui

Geshu   Geshu   Inferior angle of the scapula

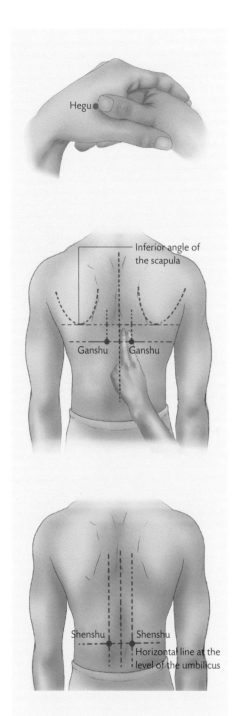

between the 1st and 2nd metacarpal bones, at the midpoint of the radial side on the 2nd metacarpal bone.

Quick location: Take the crease of the thumb interphalangeal joint of one hand and place it on the edge of the web between the thumb and forefinger of the other hand, where the tip of the thumb lands is Hegu acupoint.

Procedure: Insert the needle perpendicularly or obliquely into a depth of 0.5 to 1 cun, retaining it for 20 to 30 minutes.

Liver-Kidney Deficiency: Main Acupoints + Ganshu, Shenshu

1. Ganshu Acupoint

Location: On the back, below the spinous process of the 9th thoracic vertebra, 1.5 cun lateral to the posterior midline.

Quick location: 2 vertebrae below the intersection of the horizontal line drawn from the inferior angle of the scapula and the spine (the spinous process of the 7th thoracic vertebra), 2-finger width lateral to the lower edge.

Procedure: Insert the needle obliquely into a depth of 0.5 to 0.8 cun, retaining it for 20 to 30 minutes.

2. Shenshu Acupoint

Location: In the lumbar region, below the spinous process of the 2nd lumbar vertebra, 1.5 cun lateral to the posterior midline.

Quick location: 2-finger width lateral to the intersection of the horizontal line at the level of the umbilicus and the spine.

Procedure: Insert the needle obliquely into a depth of 0.5 to 0.8 cun, retaining it for 20 to 30 minutes.

Physician's advice: ① External application of massage, blood circulation-promoting ointments, or medicinal wine can be beneficial. ② Stiff neck can exacerbate the condition. ③ Individuals who sit for extended periods or frequently look down should take precautions to protect their cervical spine.

Stiff Neck

A stiff neck manifests as abrupt neck pain and limited mobility, often accompanied by notable tenderness in the upper back or neck and shoulder regions. It primarily denotes acute, uncomplicated neck discomfort, falling under the spectrum of neck muscle injuries. The pathological focus of this condition is in the neck and nape's muscles and meridians, and acupuncture is utilized to clear and activate collaterals, and relieve rigidity of muscle and pain. Nonetheless, recurrent occurrences of stiff neck warrant consideration of cervical spondylosis.

The main acupuncture points include Tianzhu, Houxi, Xuanzhong, Wailaogong, and Ashi. Specific acupuncture points for different patterns are as follows:

Patterns	Diagnostic Features	Acupuncture Points
Governor Vessel and Taiyang Meridian pattern	Severe pain in the neck and upper back, exacerbated by forward head bending, along with pronounced tenderness in the neck and upper back	Main acupoints + Dazhui, Shenmai
Shaoyang Meridian pattern	Neck and shoulder pain, with the head tilted towards the affected side, and notable tenderness present in the neck and shoulder region	Main acupoints + Fengchi, Jianjing

Procedure: The acupuncture technique involves lifting-thrusting reducing method, or twirling reducing method. Start by needling the distal acupuncture points while continuously twirling the needle, instructing the patient to slowly move shoulders and neck. Then needle the local acupuncture points.

Position: Prone position.

Main Acupoints

1. Tianzhu Acupoint

Location: On the nape, in the depression of the posterior hairline lateral to the trapezius muscle, approximately 1.3 cun lateral to the midline of the posterior hairline.

Quick location: Sit upright with the head lowered. Palpate the outer edge of the two major tendons on the posterior neck. The depression at this edge of the posterior hairline marks the location of this acupuncture point.

Procedure: Insert the needle perpendicularly or obliquely into a depth of 0.5 to 0.8 cun. Avoid inward and upward needle insertion to prevent injury to the medulla

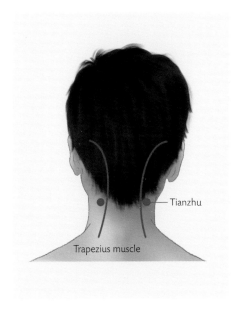

Tianzhu

Trapezius muscle

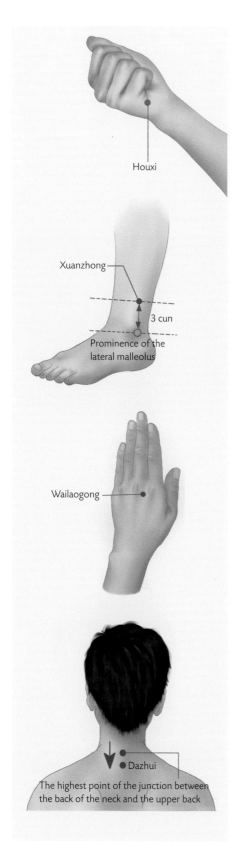

Houxi

Xuanzhong

3 cun

Prominence of the
lateral malleolus

Wailaogong

Dazhui

The highest point of the junction between
the back of the neck and the upper back

oblongata. Retain the needle for 20 to 30 minutes.

2. Houxi Acupoint

Location: On the ulnar side of the palm, with a slight fist, at the posterior margin of the 5th metacarpophalangeal joint, at the junction of the red and white flesh on the ulnar side of the palmar crease.

Procedure: Insert the needle perpendicularly or obliquely into a depth of 0.5 to 1 cun, retaining it for 20 to 30 minutes.

3. Xuanzhong Acupoint

Location: On the lateral aspect of the lower leg, 3 cun (4-finger width) above the prominence of the lateral malleolus on the anterior edge of the fibula.

Procedure: Insert the needle perpendicularly or obliquely into a depth of 0.5 to 1 cun, retaining it for 20 to 30 minutes.

4. Wailaogong Acupoint

Location: On the dorsum of the hand, between the 2nd and 3rd metacarpal bones, 0.5 cun behind the metacarpophalangeal joint.

Procedure: Insert the needle perpendicularly or obliquely into a depth of 0.5 to 0.8 cun, retaining it for 20 to 30 minutes.

5. Ashi Acupoint

Location: The tender point serves as the acupuncture point, meaning the needle is inserted directly at the site of pain.

Procedure: Insert the needle perpendicularly or obliquely into a depth of 0.5 to 1 cun, retaining it for 20 to 30 minutes.

Governing Vessel and Taiyang Meridian Pattern: Main Acupoints + Dazhui, Shenmai

1. Dazhui Acupoint

Location: In the spinal area, below the spinous process of the 7th cervical vertebra, on the posterior midline.

Quick location: Lower the head, and the

highest point of the junction between the back of the neck and the upper back corresponds to the spinous process of the 7th cervical vertebra, and the depression below it is the Dazhui acupoint.

Procedure: Insert the needle perpendicularly or obliquely into a depth of 0.5 to 1 cun, retaining it for 20 to 30 minutes.

2. Shenmai Acupoint

Location: On the lateral aspect of the foot, in the depression below the prominence of the lateral malleolus.

Procedure: Insert the needle perpendicularly or obliquely into a depth of 0.5 to 1 cun, retaining it for 20 to 30 minutes.

Shaoyang Meridian Pattern: Main Acupoints + Fengchi, Jianjing

1. Fengchi Acupoint

Location: In the posterior neck region, below the occipital bone, in the depression between the upper end of the sternocleidomastoid muscle and the trapezius muscle.

Quick location: Sit upright, and the acupoint is situated in the depression on the lateral edge of the two major tendons below the occipital bone, level with the earlobe.

Procedure: Insert the needle obliquely towards the tip of the nose with the tip of the needle slightly downward, into a depth of 0.5 to 0.8 cun, or insert the needle horizontally towards the Fengfu point (see page 133), retaining it for 20 to 30 minutes.

2. Jianjing Acupoint

Location: In the shoulder, at the midpoint of the line connecting the Dazhui acupoint and the highest point of the shoulder (acromion).

Procedure: Insert the needle obliquely upward into a depth of 0.5 to 0.8 cun, retaining it for 20 to 30 minutes.

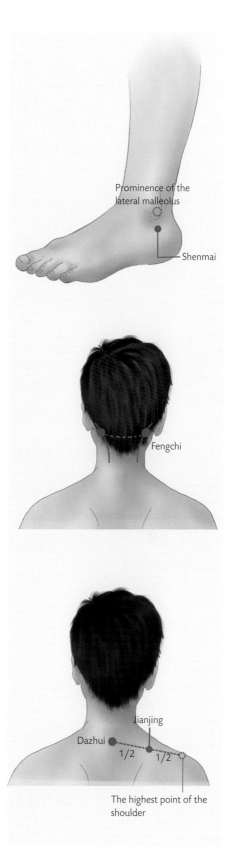

Prominence of the lateral malleolus

Shenmai

Fengchi

Jianjing

Dazhui

1/2   1/2

The highest point of the shoulder

Acute Lumbar Sprain

Acute lumbar sprain, also known as sudden tearing injuries of soft tissues like muscles, fascia, and ligaments in the lumbar region due to excessive traction from external forces, manifests with sudden onset of lower back pain, redness, or bruising of the skin at the injury site, and limited mobility. The pathological focus of this condition is in the lumbar muscles, and acupuncture treatment focuses on clearing and activating collaterals, and relieving rigidity of muscle and pain.

Acupuncture points: Yaotongdian, Weizhong, Houxi, Ashi.

Procedure: The acupuncture technique involves the lifting-thrusting reducing method or twirling reducing method. Generally, it is advisable to first needle the distal acupuncture points, and coordinate with the waist movement.

Position: Prone position.

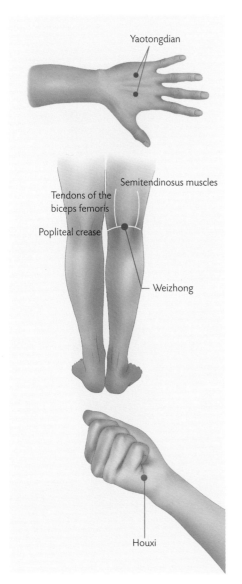

Yaotongdian

Semitendinosus muscles

Tendons of the biceps femoris

Popliteal crease

Weizhong

Houxi

1. Yaotongdian Acupoint

Location: On the dorsum of the hand, between the 2nd and 3rd metacarpal bones and the 4th and 5th metacarpal bones, at the midpoint between the dorsal wrist crease and the metacarpophalangeal joint. There are a total of four points on both hands.

Procedure: Insert the needle obliquely towards the center of the palm from both sides, into a depth of 0.5 to 0.8 cun, retaining it for 20 to 30 minutes.

2. Weizhong Acupoint

Location: In the posterior knee area, at the midpoint of the popliteal crease, between the tendons of the biceps femoris and semitendinosus muscles.

Procedure: Utilize the lifting-thrusting reducing method, and insert the needle perpendicularly into a depth of 1 to 1.5 cun, inducing limb twitching; retain the needle for 20 to 30 minutes.

3. Houxi Acupoint

Location: On the ulnar side of the palm, with a slight fist, at the posterior margin of the 5th metacarpophalangeal joint, at the junction of the red and white flesh on the ulnar side of the palmar crease.

Procedure: Insert the needle perpendicularly or obliquely into a depth of

0.5 to 1 cun, retaining it for 20 to 30 minutes.

4. Ashi Acupoint

Location: The tender point in the lumbar region serves as the acupuncture point, meaning the needle is inserted directly at the site of pain.

Procedure: Insert the needle perpendicularly or obliquely into a depth of 0.5 to 0.8 cun, retaining it for 20 to 30 minutes.

Physician's advice: ① Be mindful of protecting the lumbar region in everyday activities, especially when lifting heavy objects. ② Consider combining moving needling techniques for optimal therapeutic results. This involves needling first, followed by active or passive movements to enhance the circulation of *qi* and blood in the affected area.

Wrist Sprain

Wrist sprain refers to damage to the soft tissues around the wrist, excluding fractures, dislocations, or skin and muscle injuries. Its primary symptoms include swelling and pain in the wrist, purplish discoloration of the skin at the injury site, restricted movement of the wrist joint, and often localized warmth and discomfort. The pathological focus of this condition is in the tendon of the wrist, and acupuncture treatment focuses on improving blood circulation and alleviating stasis. Patients should avoid excessive strain on the wrist and take precautions to shield it from cold temperatures.

Acupuncture points: Yangchi, Yangxi, Yanggu, Ashi.

Procedure: The procedure may manipulate with intradermal needle or indwelling needle, which are specially designed small needles for securely placing either intradermally or subcutaneously for an extended duration.

Position: Sitting position.

1. Yangchi Acupoint

Location: Within the dorsal wrist crease, in the depression along the ulnar side (little finger side) of the extensor digitorum communis tendon.

Quick location: Hang the wrist downwards, and from the dorsal aspect of the 4th metacarpal bone, move upwards towards the crease of the wrist joint, identifying a depression that corresponds to this acupuncture point.

Procedure: Insert the needle perpendicularly or obliquely into a depth of 0.3 to 0.5 cun, retaining it for 20 to 30 minutes.

2. Yangxi Acupoint

Location: On the outer side of the dorsal wrist crease, in the depression between the

● Yangchi

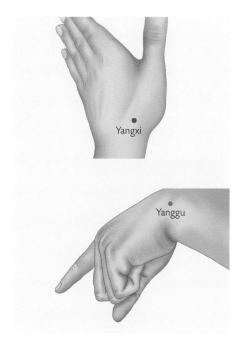

extensor digitorum longus tendon and the extensor digitorum brevis tendon of the thumb (two major tendons) when the thumb is raised.

Procedure: Insert the needle perpendicularly or obliquely into a depth of 0.3 to 0.5 cun, retaining it for 20 to 30 minutes.

3. Yanggu Acupoint

Location: On the ulnar side of the wrist, in the depression between the styloid process of the ulna and the triangular bone.

Quick location: Flex the wrist, and identify the acupoint in the depression between the two bones on the back of the wrist near the side of the little finger.

Procedure: Insert the needle perpendicularly or obliquely into a depth of 0.3 to 0.5 cun, retaining it for 20 to 30 minutes.

4. Ashi Acupoint

Location: The tender point on the wrist serves as the acupuncture point, meaning the needle is inserted directly at the site of pain.

Procedure: Insert the needle perpendicularly or obliquely into a depth of 0.3 to 0.5 cun, retaining it for 20 to 30 minutes.

Ankle Sprain

Ankle sprain, resulting from soft tissue ligament injury, manifests as swelling, pain, purplish skin, and restricted joint movement in the ankle joint. The pathological focus of this condition is in the ankle meridians, and acupuncture treatment focuses on relieving rigidity of muscle and activating collaterals, reducing swelling and alleviating pain.

The main acupuncture points for treating this condition are Shenmai, Qiuxu, Yanglao, and Ashi. Specific acupuncture points for different patterns are as follows:

Patterns	Diagnostic Features	Acupuncture Points
Taiyang Meridian of Foot	Pain on the inferior aspect of the lateral malleolus	Main acupoints + Weizhong
Shaoyang Meridian of Foot	Pain on the anterior and inferior aspect of the lateral malleolus	Main acupoints + Xuanzhong
Shaoyin Meridian of Foot	Pain on the inferior aspect of the medial malleolus	Main acupoints + Ran'gu
Taiyin Meridian of Foot	Pain on the anterior and inferior aspect of the medial malleolus	Main acupoints + Shangqiu

Procedure: Utilize lifting-thrusting reducing method or twirling reducing method. Generally, it is advisable to first needle the distal acupuncture points, and coordinate with the ankle movement.

Position: Sitting position.

Main Acupoints

1. Shenmai Acupoint

Location: On the lateral aspect of the foot, in the depression below the prominence of the lateral malleolus.

Procedure: Insert the needle perpendicularly into a depth of 0.3 to 0.5 cun, retaining it for 20 to 30 minutes.

2. Qiuxu Acupoint

Location: On the anterior and inferior aspect of the lateral malleolus, in the depression on the lateral aspect of the extensor digitorum longus tendon (the tendon that becomes visible when the 2nd to 5th toes are extended upwards).

Quick location: On the anterior and inferior aspect of the lateral malleolus, at the intersection of a vertical line dropped from the anterior edge of the lateral malleolus and a horizontal line drawn from its lower edge, in the depression.

Procedure: Insert the needle perpendicularly into a depth of 1 to 1.5 cun, retaining it for 20 to 30 minutes.

3. Yanglao Acupoint

Location: On the dorsum of the forearm, on the ulnar side (little finger side), in the depression on the proximal end of the ulnar head near the radius.

Quick location: With one hand palm-down, flat against the thorax, use the index finger of the other hand to point at the bone protruding above the wrist joint. Rotate the palm of the hand facing down towards the thorax, and the index finger will slide into the gap between the bones, identifying the Yanglao acupoint.

Procedure: Insert the needle perpendicularly into a depth of 0.5 to 0.8 cun, retaining it for 20 to 30 minutes.

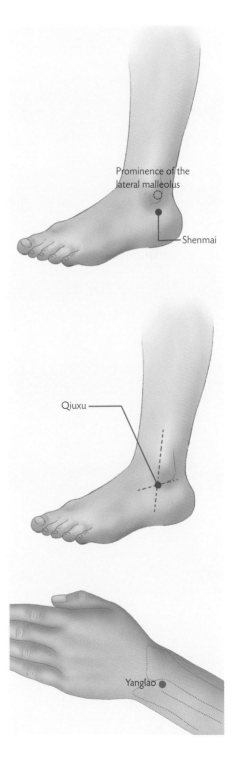

Prominence of the lateral malleolus

Shenmai

Qiuxu

Yanglao

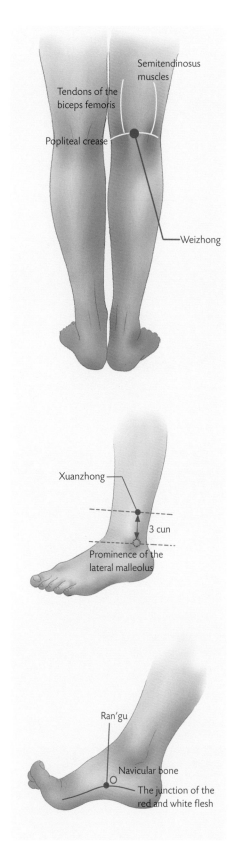

Semitendinosus
muscles

Tendons of the
biceps femoris

Popliteal crease

Weizhong

Xuanzhong

3 cun

Prominence of the
lateral malleolus

Ran'gu

Navicular bone

The junction of the
red and white flesh

4. Ashi Acupoint

Location: The tender point serves as the acupuncture point, meaning the needle is inserted directly at the site of pain.

Procedure: Insert the needle perpendicularly or obliquely into a depth of 0.5 to 0.8 cun, retaining it for 20 to 30 minutes.

Taiyang Meridian of Foot: Main Acupoints + Weizhong

Weizhong Acupoint

Location: In the posterior knee area, at the midpoint of the popliteal crease, between the tendons of the biceps femoris and semitendinosus muscles.

Procedure: Utilize the lifting-thrusting reducing method, and insert the needle perpendicularly into a depth of 1 to 1.5 cun, inducing limb twitching; retain the needle for 20 to 30 minutes.

Shaoyang Meridian of Foot: Main Acupoints + Xuanzhong

Xuanzhong Acupoint

Location: On the lateral aspect of the lower leg, 3 cun (4-finger width) above the prominence of the lateral malleolus on the anterior edge of the fibula.

Procedure: Insert the needle perpendicularly into a depth of 1 to 1.5 cun, retaining it for 20 to 30 minutes.

Shaoyin Meridian of Foot: Main Acupoints + Ran'gu

Ran'gu Acupoint

Location: On the medial edge of the foot, at the junction of the red and white flesh below the tuberosity of the navicular bone, pressing it causes a sensation of soreness and swelling.

Quick location: Find the prominent bony mark known as the navicular bone on the anterior and inferior aspect of the medial malleolus, and the acupoint is located in the depression anterior and inferior to the bone.

Procedure: Insert the needle perpendicularly into a depth of 0.5 to 1 cun, retaining it for 20 to 30 minutes.

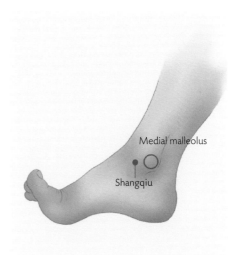

Taiyin Meridian of Foot: Main Acupoints + Shangqiu

Shangqiu Acupoint

Location: In the depression on the anterior and inferior aspect of the medial malleolus of the foot.

Procedure: Insert the needle perpendicularly into a depth of 0.5 to 0.8 cun, retaining it for 20 to 30 minutes.

 Physician's advice: ① Restrict foot movement appropriately after injury to prevent exacerbating the condition. ② Apply cold compress in the early stage of the sprain, and switch to hot compress after 24 hours. ③ Moxibustion with warming needle can commence on the second day, with each session lasting about 20 minutes. The specific duration can be determined based on the patient's condition. Once the swelling subsides, conventional needle insertion methods can be adopted.

Lumbago

The primary symptom is lumbar pain, with its underlying mechanism involving obstruction of the lumbar meridians, blockade of blood and *qi*, or deficiency of kidney essence, leading to insufficient nourishment and warmth in the lumbar region. Acupuncture treatment focuses on facilitating meridian circulation and alleviating pain.

The main acupuncture points include Shenshu, Dachangshu, Weizhong, Yaojiaji, and Ashi. Specific acupuncture points for different patterns are as follows:

Patterns	Diagnostic Features	Acupuncture Points
Lumbago with cold-damp syndrome	Cold, heavy sensation in the lumbar region worsened by rainy or cold weather; pale tongue with a white, slippery coating	Main acupoints + Yaoyangguan
Lumbago with static blood syndrome	Mostly with history of trauma, fixed stabbing pain in the waist area; dark tongue or presence of ecchymosis	Main acupoints + Geshu
Lumbago with kidney deficiency syndrome	Soreness and pain in the lumbar region aggravated by exertion	Main acupoints + Taixi

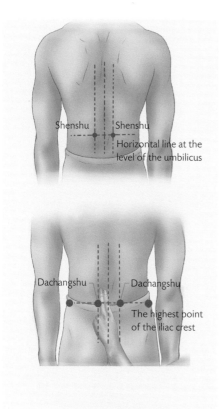

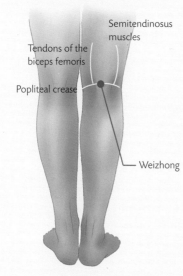

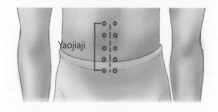

Procedure: Conventional needle insertion. For lumbago with cold-damp syndrome or lumbago with kidney deficiency syndrome, moxibustion with warming needle can be added.

Position: Prone position.

Main Acupoints

1. Shenshu Acupoint

Location: In the lumbar region, below the spinous process of the 2nd lumbar vertebra, 1.5 cun lateral to the posterior midline.

Quick location: 2-finger width lateral to the intersection of the horizontal line at the level of the umbilicus and the spine.

Procedure: Insert the needle obliquely into a depth of 0.5 to 0.8 cun, retaining it for 20 to 30 minutes.

2. Dachangshu Acupoint

Location: At the waist, below the spinous process of the 4th lumbar vertebra, 1.5 cun lateral to the posterior midline.

Quick location: 2-finger width lateral to the intersection of the spine and the line connecting the highest point of the iliac crest on both sides.

Procedure: Insert the needle obliquely into a depth of 0.5 to 0.8 cun, retaining it for 20 to 30 minutes.

3. Weizhong Acupoint

Location: In the posterior knee area, at the midpoint of the popliteal crease, between the tendons of the biceps femoris and semitendinosus muscles.

Procedure: Insert the needle perpendicularly into a depth of 1 to 1.5 cun, retaining it for 20 to 30 minutes.

4. Yaojiaji Acupoint

Location: On both sides below the spinous processes of the 1st lumbar vertebra to the 5th lumbar vertebra, 0.5 cun (half-finger width) lateral to the posterior midline.

Procedure: Insert the needle perpendicularly into a depth of 0.3 to 0.5 cun, retaining it for 20 to 30 minutes.

5. Ashi Acupoint

Location: The tender point in the lumbar region serves as the acupuncture point, meaning the needle is inserted directly at the site of pain.

Procedure: Insert the needle perpendicularly or obliquely into a depth of 0.5 to 0.8 cun, retaining it for 20 to 30 minutes.

Lumbago with Cold-Damp Syndrome: Main Acupoints + Yaoyangguan

Yaoyangguan Acupoint

Location: In the lumbar region, on the posterior midline, in the depression below the spinous process of the 4th lumbar vertebra.

Quick location: Find the point in the depression below the spinous process of the 4th lumbar vertebra, where the line connecting the highest points of the iliac crests on both sides intersects with the posterior midline of the back.

Procedure: Insert the needle obliquely upward into a depth of 1 to 1.5 cun, retaining it for 20 to 30 minutes.

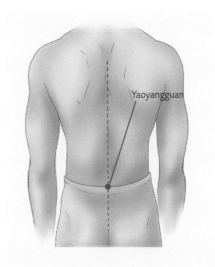

Lumbago with Static Blood Syndrome: Main Acupoints + Geshu

Geshu Acupoint

Location: On the back, below the spinous process of the 7th thoracic vertebra, 1.5 cun lateral to the posterior midline.

Quick location: The intersection of the horizontal line drawn from the inferior angle of the scapula and the spine (the spinous process of the 7th thoracic vertebra), 2-finger width lateral to the lower edge.

Procedure: Insert the needle perpendicularly into a depth of 0.5 to 1 cun, retaining it for 20 to 30 minutes.

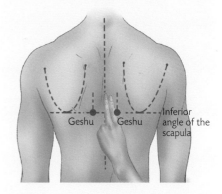

Lumbago with Kidney Deficiency Syndrome: Main Acupoints + Taixi

Taixi Acupoint

Location: On the medial aspect of the foot, in the depression between the prominence of the

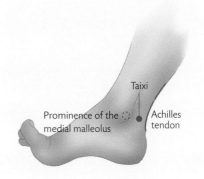

lateral malleolus and the Achilles tendon.

Procedure: Insert the needle perpendicularly into a depth of 0.5 to 0.8 cun, retaining it for 20 to 30 minutes.

 Physician's advice: ① Avoid prolonged sitting without movement. ② Enhance daily exercise and cultivate proper walking posture and demeanor to prevent excessive strain in the lumbar region.

Shoulder Periarthritis

Shoulder periarthritis, characterized by shoulder pain with fixed site, and limited movement, often exacerbated by weather changes or fatigue, particularly at night, is more prevalent in adults around the age of 50. The pathological focus of this condition is in the shoulder muscles, and acupuncture treatment focuses on activating meridians and relieving rigidity of muscle and pain.

The main acupuncture points include Jianyu, Jianliao, Jianzhen, Jianqian, Yanglingquan, Tiaokou, and Ashi. Specific acupuncture points for different patterns are as follows:

Patterns	Diagnostic Features	Acupuncture Points
Yangming Meridian of Hand	Predominant pain felt on the anterior lateral aspect of the shoulder, with pronounced tenderness upon pressure; significant pain or tenderness at the Jianyu acupoint, exacerbating during shoulder abduction	Main acupoints + Sanjian
Shaoyang Meridian of Hand	Predominant pain felt on the lateral aspect of the shoulder, with pronounced tenderness upon pressure; significant pain or tenderness at the Jianliao acupoint, exacerbating during shoulder abduction.	Main acupoints + Zhongzhu
Taiyang Meridian of Hand	Predominant pain felt on the posterior aspect of the shoulder, with pronounced tenderness upon pressure; significant pain or tenderness at the Jianzhen and Naoshu acupoints, exacerbating during shoulder adduction	Main acupoints + Houxi
Taiyin Meridian of Hand	Predominant pain felt on the anterior aspect of the shoulder, with pronounced tenderness upon pressure, exacerbating when extending the shoulder backwards	Main acupoints + Lieque

Procedure: Utilize the lifting-thrusting reducing method, twirling reducing method, or even reinforcing-reducing method. First needle the distal acupuncture points, and coordinate with the shoulder joint movement after insertion.

Position: Sitting position.

Main Acupoints

1. Jianyu Acupoint

Location: In the depression below the anterior acromion when the shoulder is abduced or stretched forwards.

Procedure: Insert the needle perpendicularly or obliquely upward into a depth of 0.8 to 1.5 cun, retaining it for 20 to 30 minutes.

2. Jianliao Acupoint

Location: In the depression below the posterior acromion when the arm is abduced.

Procedure: Insert the needle perpendicularly into a depth of 1 to 1.5 cun, retaining it for 20 to 30 minutes.

3. Jianzhen Acupoint

Location: 1 cun (1-finger width) above the posterior axillary fold when the arm is adducted.

Procedure: Insert the needle perpendicularly into a depth of 1 to 1.5 cun, retaining it for 20 to 30 minutes.

4. Jianqian Acupoint

Location: Sit upright with relaxed shoulders, and identify the midpoint between the apex of the anterior axillary fold and the Jianyu acupoint.

Procedure: Insert the needle perpendicularly or obliquely upward into a depth of 0.8 to 1.5 cun, retaining it for 20 to 30 minutes.

5. Yanglingquan Acupoint

Location: On the lateral aspect of the lower leg, in the depression below the anterior capitulum fibulae.

Procedure: Insert the needle perpendicularly or obliquely into a depth of 0.5 to 1 cun, retaining it for 20 to 30 minutes.

6. Tiaokou Acupoint

Location: On the anterior-lateral aspect of the lower leg, 8 cun below the Dubi acupoint and 1-finger width from the anterior border of the tibia.

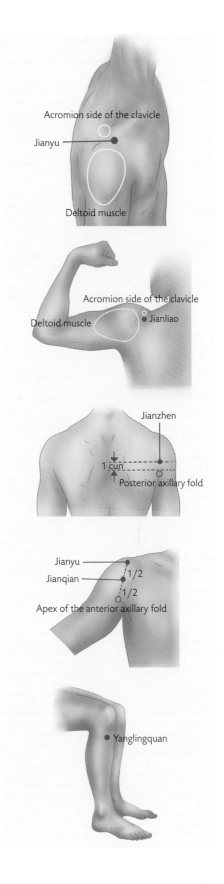

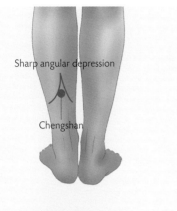

Sharp angular depression

Chengshan

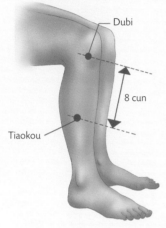

Dubi

8 cun

Tiaokou

Procedure: Insert the needle perpendicularly towards the Chengshan acupoint from the Tiaokou acupoint into a depth of 1 to 2 cun, retaining it for 20 to 30 minutes. (Chengshan acupoint is situated in the sharp angular depression beneath the belly of the gastrocnemius muscle when the lower leg is extended or the heel is raised.)

7. Ashi Acupoint

Location: The tender point serves as the acupuncture point, meaning the needle is inserted directly at the site of pain.

Procedure: Insert the needle perpendicularly or obliquely into a depth of 0.5 to 1 cun, retaining it for 20 to 30 minutes.

Yangming Meridian of Hand: Main Acupoints + Sanjian

Sanjian Acupoint

Location: With a slight fist clench, in the depression behind the 2nd metacarpophalangeal joint on the radial side of the index finger (towards the thumb side).

Procedure: Insert the needle perpendicularly into a depth of 0.3 to 0.5 cun, retaining it for 20 to 30 minutes.

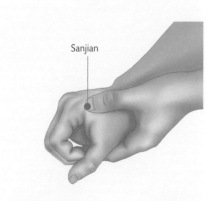

Sanjian

Shaoyang Meridian of Hand: Main Acupoints + Zhongzhu

Zhongzhu Acupoint

Location: On the dorsum of the hand, behind the 4th metacarpophalangeal joint, in the depression between the 4th and 5th metacarpal bones.

Procedure: Insert the needle perpendicularly or obliquely into a depth of 0.5 to 0.8 cun, retaining it for 20 to 30 minutes.

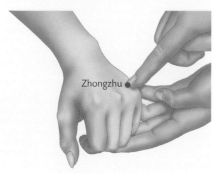

Zhongzhu

Taiyang Meridian of Hand: Main Acupoints + Houxi

Houxi Acupoint

Location: On the ulnar side of the palm, with

a slight fist, at the posterior margin of the 5th metacarpophalangeal joint, at the junction of the red and white flesh on the ulnar side of the palmar crease.

Procedure: Insert the needle perpendicularly or obliquely into a depth of 0.5 to 1 cun, retaining it for 20 to 30 minutes.

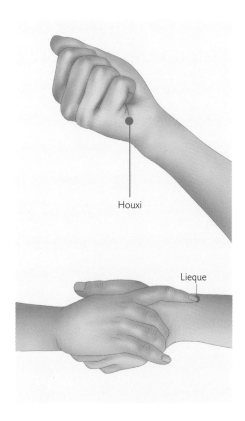

Houxi

Lieque

Taiyin Meridian of Hand: Main Acupoints + Lieque

Lieque Acupoint

Location: Cross the hands naturally with the tiger's mouth of hand, and press one index finger on the styloid process of the radius (the high prominence on the thumb side behind the wrist). The acupuncture point is located under the fingertip of the index finger.

Procedure: Insert the needle perpendicularly or obliquely into a depth of 0.5 to 1 cun, retaining it for 20 to 30 minutes.

 Physician's advice: ① If there is no relief after an extended treatment duration, consider other underlying conditions. ② During the treatment, patients should engage in suitable shoulder joint functional exercises and pay attention to keeping the shoulder area warm.

Elbow Pain

Elbow pain is characterized by discomfort during elbow joint movement, which may radiate to the forearm, wrist, and upper limb. Its onset is typically gradual and recurrent without clear trauma. While local swelling and pain may not be obvious, there are distinct but non-fixed tender points. Elbow joint movement remains unrestricted. This condition is more prevalent among individuals engaged in activities involving frequent rotation of the forearm and flexion and extension of the elbow joint. The pathological focus of this condition is on the elbow, specifically the three *yang* meridians of the hand. Acupuncture treatment focuses on activating collaterals and relieving rigidity of muscle and pain.

The main acupuncture points include Quchi, Zhouliao, Yanglingquan, and Ashi. Specific acupuncture points for different patterns are as follows:

Patterns	Diagnostic Features	Acupuncture Points
Yangming Meridian of Hand	Obvious tenderness point above the lateral upper part of the elbow joint	Main acupoints + Shousanli, Sanjian
Taiyang Meridian of Hand	Obvious tenderness point below the medial lower part of the elbow joint	Main acupoints + Xiaohai, Yanggu
Shaoyang Meridian of Hand	Obvious tenderness point on the lateral side of the elbow joint	Main acupoints + Tianjing, Waiguan

Procedure: Utilize lifting-thrusting reducing method or twirling reducing method. Start by needling the tender point opposite to the Yanglingquan acupoint while concurrently mobilizing the affected area. Multiple points can be needled simultaneously. Additionally, warming needle moxibustion or local point moxa-cone moxibustion for 20 to 30 minutes can be incorporated as needed.

Position: Sitting position.

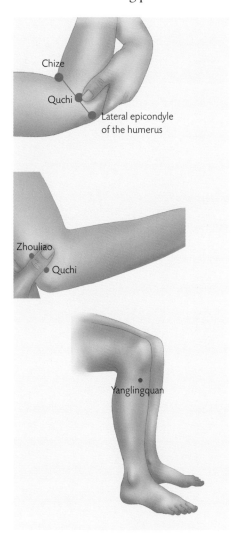

Main Acupoints

1. Quchi Acupoint

Location: At the lateral end of the cubital crease, with the elbow flexed, at the midpoint of the line connecting the Chize acupoint with the lateral epicondyle of the humerus.

Procedure: Insert the needle perpendicularly or obliquely into a depth of 0.5 to 1 cun, retaining it for 20 to 30 minutes.

2. Zhouliao Acupoint

Location: On the lateral aspect of the arm, with the elbow flexed, 1 cun (1-finger width) above the Quchi point, along the edge of the humerus.

Procedure: Insert the needle perpendicularly into a depth of 0.5 to 1 cun, retaining it for 20 to 30 minutes.

3. Yanglingquan Acupoint

Location: On the lateral aspect of the lower leg, in the depression below the anterior capitulum fibulae.

Procedure: Insert the needle perpendicularly or obliquely into a depth of 0.5 to 1 cun, retaining it for 20 to 30 minutes.

4. Ashi Acupoint

Location: The tender point serves as the acupuncture point, meaning the needle is inserted directly at the site of pain.

Procedure: Insert the needle perpendicularly or obliquely into a depth of 0.5 to 1 cun, retaining it for 20 to 30 minutes.

Yangming Meridian of Hand: Main Acupoints + Shousanli, Sanjian

1. Shousanli Acupoint

Location: On the radial side of the dorsum of the forearm, along the line connecting Yangxi acupoint and Quchi acupoint, 2 cun (3-finger width) below the cubital crease.

Procedure: Insert the needle perpendicularly into a depth of 0.5 to 1 cun, retaining it for 20 to 30 minutes.

2. Sanjian Acupoint

Location: With a slight fist clench, in the depression behind the 2nd metacarpophalangeal joint on the radial side of the index finger (towards the thumb side).

Procedure: Insert the needle perpendicularly into a depth of 0.3 to 0.5 cun, retaining it for 20 to 30 minutes.

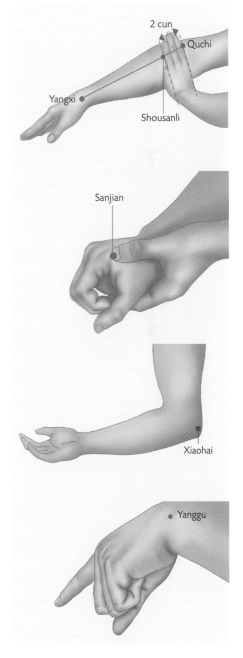

Taiyang Meridian of Hand: Main Acupoints + Xiaohai, Yanggu

1. Xiaohai Acupoint

Location: On the medial aspect of the elbow, in the depression between the olecranon process of ulna and the medial epicondyle of humerus.

Quick location: Bend the elbow joint, and locate the depression between the highest point of the elbow tip and the highest point of the protruding bone on the medial aspect of the elbow (little finger side).

Procedure: Insert the needle perpendicularly into a depth of 0.3 to 0.8 cun, retaining it for 20 to 30 minutes.

2. Yanggu Acupoint

Location: In the depression between the styloid process of the ulna and the triangular bone.

Quick location: Flex the wrist, and identify the acupoint in the depression between the two bones on the back of the wrist near the side of the little finger.

Procedure: Insert the needle

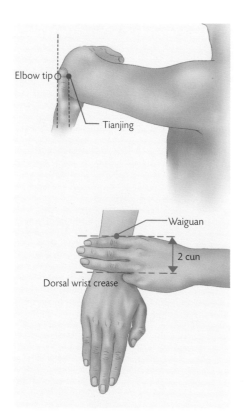

Elbow tip — Tianjing

Waiguan — 2 cun — Dorsal wrist crease

perpendicularly into a depth of 0.3 to 0.5 cun, retaining it for 20 to 30 minutes.

Shaoyang Meridian of Hand: Main Acupoints + Tianjing, Waiguan

1. Tianjing Acupoint

Location: In the depression 1 cun (1-finger width) directly above the elbow tip when the elbow is flexed.

Procedure: Insert the needle perpendicularly into a depth of 0.3 to 1 cun, retaining it for 20 to 30 minutes.

2. Waiguan Acupoint

Location: On the dorsum of the forearm, along the line connecting the Yangchi acupoint and the elbow tip, 2 cun (3-finger width) above the dorsal wrist crease, between the ulna and radius (two major bones).

Procedure: Insert the needle perpendicularly or obliquely into a depth of 0.5 to 1 cun, retaining it for 20 to 30 minutes.

Physician's advice: ① Reduce elbow joint movement and ensure local warmth during the acute phase of the patient. ② Consider using massage or applying ointments or medicinal wine with blood-activating properties for fumigation and other treatments. ③ Incorporate moving needling techniques for optimal therapeutic results. This involves needling first followed by active or passive movements to facilitate the circulation of *qi* and blood in the affected area.

Heel Pain

Heel pain, whether acute or chronic, stems from injuries affecting the foot's heel region. Key symptoms include pain in the heel and sole while standing or walking, often accompanied by reluctance to put weight on the foot. The pain may extend forward to the forefoot, intensifying during physical activity and walking, while subsiding during rest. The pathological focus of this condition is in the foot's fascia, and acupuncture treatment focuses on activating meridians and collaterals.

Acupuncture points: Zhaohai, Kunlun, Shenmai, Xuanzhong, Ashi.

Procedure: Utilize the lifting-thrusting reducing method, twirling reducing method, or even reinforcing-reducing method.

Position: Prone position.

1. Zhaohai Acupoint

Location: On the medial aspect of the foot, 1 cun below the prominence of the medial malleolus in the depression.

Procedure: Utilize the twirling reinforcing method, and insert the needle perpendicularly into a depth of 0.8 to 1.2 cun, retaining it for 20 to 30 minutes.

2. Kunlun Acupoint

Location: Posterior to the lateral malleolus, in the depression between the prominence of the lateral malleolus and the Achilles tendon.

Procedure: Insert the needle perpendicularly into a depth of 0.5 to 0.8 cun, retaining it for 20 to 30 minutes.

3. Shenmai Acupoint

Location: In the depression below the prominence of the lateral malleolus.

Procedure: Insert the needle perpendicularly or obliquely into a depth of 0.5 to 1 cun, retaining it for 20 to 30 minutes.

4. Xuanzhong Acupoint

Location: On the lateral aspect of the lower leg, 3 cun above the prominence of the lateral malleolus on the anterior edge of the fibula.

Procedure: Insert the needle perpendicularly or obliquely into a depth of 0.5 to 1 cun, retaining it for 20 to 30 minutes.

5. Ashi Acupoint

Location: The tender point serves as the acupuncture point, meaning the needle is inserted directly at the site of pain.

Procedure: Insert the needle perpendicularly or obliquely into a depth of 0.5 to 1 cun, retaining it for 20 to 30 minutes.

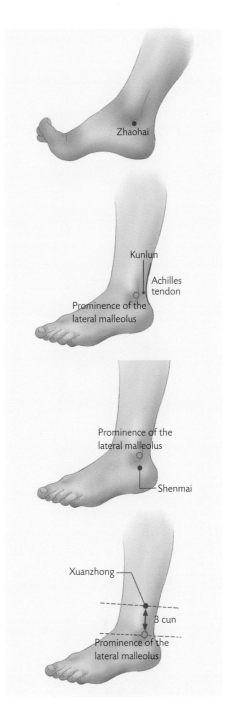

Physician's advice: ① Acute patients should prioritize rest, and gradually reduce standing or walking time as symptoms alleviate. ② It is advisable to wear soft-soled shoes regularly or place sponge pads inside the shoes on the affected foot. ③ Maintain a balance between activity and rest, and avoid exposure to windy, cold, or damp conditions.

CHAPTER SIX
Acupuncture Treatment for Gynecological Conditions

T his chapter covers common gynecological conditions such as menstrual disorders, dysmenorrhea, and issues faced by women during special periods, including menopausal syndrome and insufficient lactation. It is essential to note that acupuncture should be performed by a professional; caution is advised, and acupuncture intensity should be within the patient's tolerance.

Menstrual Disorders

Menstrual disorders are characterized by abnormalities in the menstrual cycle, flow, color, and property. Clinical presentations include advanced menstruation, retarded menstruation and irregular menstrual cycle. The pathological focus of this condition is in the uterus.

Specific acupuncture points for different patterns are as follows:

Patterns	Diagnostic Features	Acupuncture Points
Advanced menstruation	Menstruation onset 1 to 2 weeks earlier, persisting for more than two menstrual cycles	Guanyuan, Xuehai, Sanyinjiao
Retarded menstruation	Menstruation onset 1 to 2 weeks later, or occurring once every 3 to 5 months, persisting for more than two menstrual cycles	Qihai, Guilai, Sanyinjiao
Irregular menstrual cycle	Menstruation onset 1 to 2 weeks earlier or later, persisting for more than three menstrual cycles	Guanyuan, Sanyinjiao

Procedure: Conventional needle insertion.
Position: Lateral position.

Advanced Menstruation

1. Guanyuan Acupoint
Location: In the lower abdomen, on the anterior midline, 3 cun (4-finger width) below the umbilicus.
Procedure: Insert the needle obliquely downward into a depth of 1.5 to 2 cun, retaining it for 20 to 30 minutes.

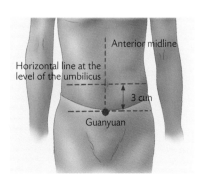

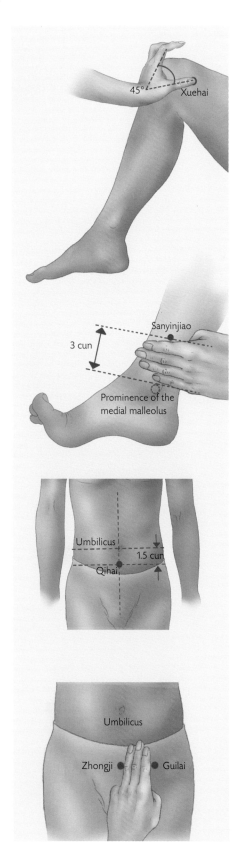

2. Xuehai Acupoint

Location: Bend the knee; on the medial aspect of the thigh, 2 cun above the medial end of the base of patella, at the medial prominence of the quadriceps femoris muscle.

Quick location: Place the left (right) palm directly above the upper edge of the right (left) kneecap on the inner side of the thigh. Extend the 2nd to 5th fingers upward in a straight line, while maintaining a 45° angle between the thumb and the other four fingers. The acupoint is just beneath the tip of the thumb.

Procedure: Insert the needle perpendicularly into a depth of 1 to 1.5 cun, retaining it for 20 to 30 minutes.

3. Sanyinjiao Acupoint

Location: On the medial aspect of the lower leg, 3 cun (4-finger width) above the prominence of the medial malleolus, posterior to the medial border of the tibia.

Procedure: Insert the needle perpendicularly into a depth of 1 to 1.5 cun, retaining it for 20 to 30 minutes (contraindicated during pregnancy).

Retarded Menstruation

1. Qihai Acupoint

Location: In the lower abdomen, on the anterior midline, 1.5 cun (about 2-finger width) below the umbilicus.

Procedure: Insert the needle obliquely downward into a depth of 1 to 1.5 cun, retaining it for 20 to 30 minutes.

2. Guilai Acupoint

Location: 4 cun (5-finger width) below the umbilicus, 2 cun (3-finger width) lateral to the anterior midline, precisely below the nipple.

Procedure: Insert the needle perpendicularly into a depth of 1 to 1.5 cun, retaining the needle for 20 to 30 minutes.

3. Sanyinjiao Acupoint

Location: On the medial aspect of the lower leg, 3 cun (4-finger width) above the prominence of the medial malleolus, posterior to the medial border of the tibia.

Procedure: Insert the needle perpendicularly into a depth of 1 to 1.5 cun, retaining it for 20 to 30 minutes (contraindicated during pregnancy).

Irregular Menstrual Cycle

1. Guanyuan Acupoint

Location: In the lower abdomen, on the anterior midline, 3 cun (4-finger width) below the umbilicus.

Procedure: Insert the needle obliquely into a depth of 1.5 to 2 cun, retaining it for 20 to 30 minutes.

2. Sanyinjiao Acupoint

Location: On the medial aspect of the lower leg, 3 cun (4-finger width) above the prominence of the medial malleolus, posterior to the medial border of the tibia.

Procedure: Insert the needle perpendicularly into a depth of 1 to 1.5 cun, retaining it for 20 to 30 minutes (contraindicated during pregnancy).

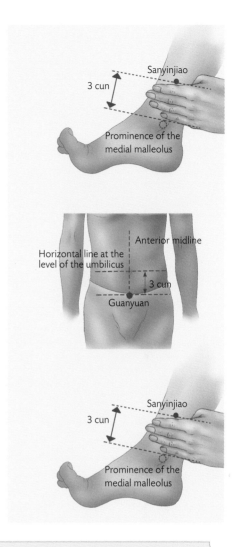

 Physician's advice: Acupuncture demonstrates favorable efficacy in treating functional menstrual disorders. However, in cases where menstrual disorders are caused by organic lesion, it is crucial to investigate and identify the underlying causes.

Dysmenorrhea

Dysmenorrhea refers to cyclical lower abdominal pain that occurs during or around menstruation. The pathological focus of this condition is in the uterus and can be categorized into three patterns: *qi* stagnation, cold coagulation, and deficiency. Acupuncture treatment is centered on coordinating Thoroughfare and Conception Vessels, and warming the meridians for alleviating pain.

The main acupuncture points are Zhongji, Sanyinjiao, Diji, and Ciliao. Specific acupuncture points for different patterns are as follows:

Patterns	Diagnostic Features	Acupuncture Points
Qi stagnation	Mainly characterized by distending pain, with major discomfort in the chest, hypochondrium, and breasts; blood clots may be present during menstruation; tongue may exhibit ecchymosis or petechiae	Main acupoints + Taichong, Xuehai
Cold coagulation	Mainly characterized by cold pain, which alleviates with warmth	Main acupoints + Guanyuan, Guilai
Physical weakness	Pain is relieved by pressing	Main acupoints + Qihai, Shenshu

Procedure: Insert a needle at Zhongji acupoint, using a continuous twirling method to guide the needle sensation downward. Conventional needle insertion is applied for other acupoints.

Position: Prone position.

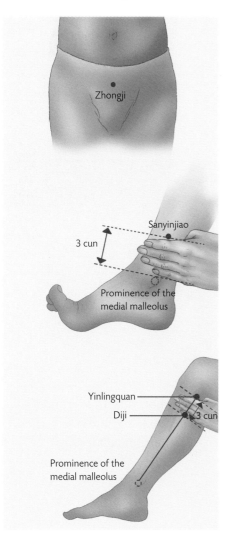

Main Acupoints

1. Zhongji Acupoint

Location: In the lower abdomen, on the anterior midline, 4 cun below the umbilicus.

Quick location: 1-finger width below Guanyuan acupoint (see page 119).

Procedure: Insert the needle perpendicularly into a depth of 1 to 1.5 cun, retaining it for 20 to 30 minutes.

2. Sanyinjiao Acupoint

Location: On the medial aspect of the lower leg, 3 cun (4-finger width) above the prominence of the medial malleolus, posterior to the medial border of the tibia.

Procedure: Insert the needle perpendicularly into a depth of 1 to 1.5 cun, retaining it for 20 to 30 minutes (contraindicated during pregnancy).

3. Diji Acupoint

Location: On the medial aspect of the lower leg, on the line between Yinlingquan acupoint and the prominence of the medial malleolus, 3 cun (4-finger width) below the Yinlingquan acupoint.

Procedure: Insert the needle perpendicularly into a depth of 1 to 1.5 cun, retaining it for 20 to 30 minutes.

4. Ciliao Acupoint

Location: In the sacral region, directly opposite the 2nd posterior sacral foramen.

Procedure: Insert the needle perpendicularly into a depth of 1 to 1.5 cun, retaining it for 20 to 30 minutes.

Qi Stagnation: Main Acupoints + Taichong, Xuehai

1. Taichong Acupoint

Location: On the dorsum of the foot, at the depression in front of the junction between the 1st and 2nd metatarsal bones.

Quick location: On the dorsum of the foot, push upward along the crease between the 1st and 2nd toes. The depression felt is the Taichong acupoint.

Procedure: Insert the needle obliquely into a depth of 0.5 to 1 cun, retaining it for 20 to 30 minutes.

2. Xuehai Acupoint

Location: Bend the knee; on the medial aspect of the thigh, 2 cun above the medial end of the patella, at the medial prominence of the quadriceps femoris muscle.

Quick location: Place the left (right) palm directly above the upper edge of the right (left) kneecap on the inner side of the thigh. Extend the 2nd to 5th fingers upward in a straight line, while maintaining a 45° angle between the thumb and the other four fingers. The acupoint is just beneath the tip of the thumb.

Procedure: Insert the needle perpendicularly into a depth of 1 to 1.5 cun, retaining it for 20 to 30 minutes.

Cold Coagulation: Main Acupoints + Guanyuan, Guilai

1. Guanyuan Acupoint

Location: In the lower abdomen, on the

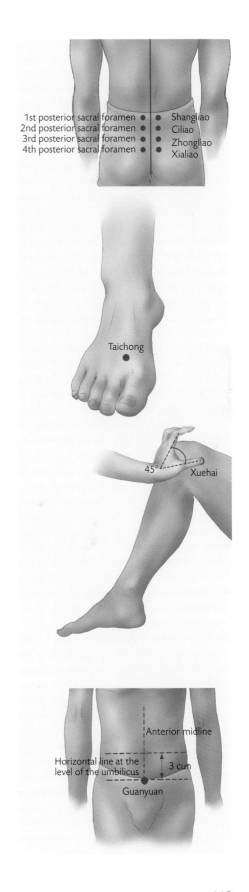

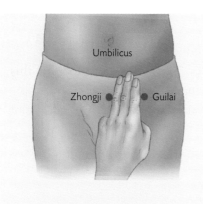

anterior midline, 3 cun (4-finger width) below the umbilicus.

Procedure: Insert the needle obliquely into a depth of 1.5 to 2 cun, retaining it for 20 to 30 minutes.

2. Guilai Acupoint

Location: 4 cun (5-finger width) below the umbilicus, 2 cun (3-finger width) lateral to the anterior midline, precisely below the nipple.

Procedure: Insert the needle perpendicularly into a depth of 1 to 1.5 cun, retaining the needle for 20 to 30 minutes.

Physical Weakness: Main Acupoints + Qihai, Shenshu

1. Qihai Acupoint

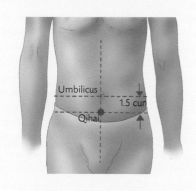

Location: In the lower abdomen, on the anterior midline, 1.5 cun (about 2-finger width) below the umbilicus.

Procedure: Insert the needle obliquely into a depth of 1 to 1.5 cun, retaining it for 20 to 30 minutes.

2. Shenshu Acupoint

Location: In the lumbar region, at the same level as the inferior border of the spinous process of the 2nd lumbar vertebra, 1.5 cun lateral to the posterior midline.

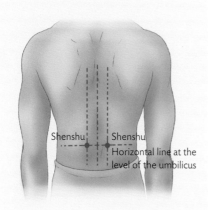

Quick location: 2-finger width lateral to the intersection of the horizontal line at the level of the umbilicus and the spine.

Procedure: Insert the needle obliquely into a depth of 0.5 to 0.8 cun, retaining it for 20 to 30 minutes.

Physician's advice: ① To prevent dysmenorrhea, initiate treatment from 3 to 7 days before the menstrual period, with a continuous treatment for three menstrual cycles as one course of therapy. ② For secondary dysmenorrhea, identify the underlying causes. ③ Pay attention to menstrual hygiene and keep warm, avoiding the consumption of cold foods, excessive stress, and overexertion.

Amenorrhea

Amenorrhea refers to the absence of menstruation in individuals aged 16 and above, or the cessation of menstruation for more than three cycles. The pathological focus of this condition is in the uterus, and the acupuncture treatment is centered on coordinating the Thoroughfare and Conception Vessels, promoting blood circulation, and facilitating menstrual flow.

Specific acupuncture points for different patterns are as follows:

Patterns	Diagnostic Features	Acupuncture Points
Amenorrhea due to blood depletion	Absence of menstruation by the age of 16 or a gradual reduction in menstrual flow until complete cessation	Guanyuan, Pishu, Shenshu, Zusanli
Amenorrhea due to blood stagnation	Amenorrhea along with emotional depression, body swelling and pain, dark and purplish tongue color, or cold pain in the lower abdomen which alleviates with warmth	Zhongji, Taichong, Sanyinjiao, Hegu

Procedure: Use lifting-thrusting reinforcing method or twirling reinforcing method for amenorrhea due to blood depletion, and lifting-thrusting reducing method or twirling reducing method for amenorrhea due to blood stagnation.

Position: Lateral position.

Amenorrhea Due to Blood Depletion

1. Guanyuan Acupoint

Location: In the lower abdomen, on the anterior midline, 3 cun (4-finger width) below the umbilicus.

Procedure: Heavy moxibustion with large moxa cones.

2. Pishu Acupoint

Location: On the back, at the same level as the inferior border of the spinous process of the 11st thoracic vertebra, 1.5 cun lateral to the posterior midline.

Quick location: 3 vertebrae above the intersection of the horizontal line at the level of the umbilicus and the spine, 2-finger width lateral to the lower border.

Procedure: Insert the needle perpendicularly or obliquely into a depth of 0.5 to 1 cun, retaining it for 20 to 30 minutes.

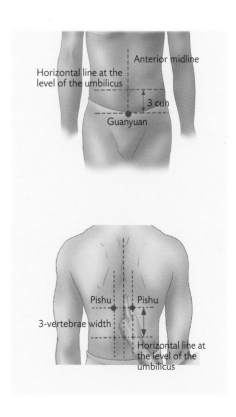

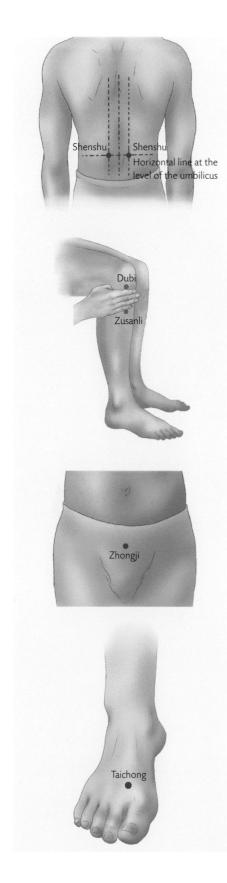

3. Shenshu Acupoint

Location: In the lumbar region, below the spinous process of the 2nd lumbar vertebra, 1.5 cun lateral to the posterior midline.

Quick location: 2-finger width lateral to the intersection of the horizontal line at the level of the umbilicus and the spine.

Procedure: Insert the needle obliquely into a depth of 0.5 to 0.8 cun, retaining it for 20 to 30 minutes.

4. Zusanli Acupoint

Location: On the lateral aspect of the lower leg, 3 cun (4-finger width) below the Dubi acupoint, 1-finger width lateral to the anterior crest of the tibia.

Quick location: Stand and bend over; use the tiger's mouth of hand on the same side to encircle the upper lateral border of the patella, with the remaining 4 fingers pointing downward, and the tip of the middle finger is this acupoint.

Procedure: Insert the needle perpendicularly or obliquely into a depth of 0.5 to 1 cun, retaining it for 20 to 30 minutes.

Amenorrhea Due to Blood Stagnation

1. Zhongji Acupoint

Location: In the lower abdomen, on the anterior midline, 4 cun below the umbilicus.

Quick location: 1-finger width below Guanyuan acupoint (see page 119).

Procedure: Insert the needle perpendicularly into a depth of 1 to 1.5 cun, retaining it for 20 to 30 minutes.

2. Taichong Acupoint

Location: On the dorsum of the foot, at the depression in front of the junction between the 1st and 2nd metatarsal bones.

Quick location: On the dorsum of the foot, push upward along the crease between the 1st and 2nd toes. The depression felt is the Taichong acupoint.

Procedure: Insert the needle perpendicularly into a depth of 0.5 to 0.8 cun, retaining it for 20 to 30 minutes.

3. Sanyinjiao Acupoint

Location: On the medial aspect of the lower leg, 3 cun (4-finger width) above the prominence of the medial malleolus, posterior to the medial border of the tibia.

Procedure: Utilizing the lifting-thrusting reinforcing method, insert the needle perpendicularly or obliquely into a depth of 0.5 to 1 cun, retaining it for 20 to 30 minutes (contraindicated during pregnancy).

4. Hegu Acupoint

Location: On the back of the hand, between the 1st and 2nd metacarpal bones, at the midpoint of the radial side on the 2nd metacarpal bone.

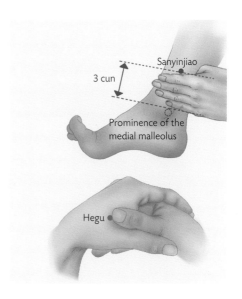

Quick location: Take the crease of thumb interphalangeal joint of one hand and place it on the edge of the web between the thumb and forefinger of the other hand, where the tip of the thumb lands is Hegu acupoint.

Procedure: Insert the needle perpendicularly or obliquely into a depth of 0.5 to 1 cun, retaining it for 20 to 30 minutes.

 Physician's advice: ① Pregnancy should be ruled out first when experiencing amenorrhea. ② Prior to treatment, relevant examinations should be conducted to identify the root cause of the condition.

Menopausal Syndrome

Menopausal syndrome refers to a set of symptoms that occur before and after menopause, with the main manifestations being menstrual cessation or disorders, depression, irritability, and hot flashes with sweating. The pathological focus of this condition is in the kidneys. Acupuncture treatment focuses on nourishing kidney essence and coordinating the Thoroughfare and Conception Vessels. Patients also need to relax and maintain a positive mindset.

Acupuncture points: Guanyuan, Sanyinjiao, Shenshu, Taixi.

Procedure: Utilize the lifting-thrusting reinforcing method, twirling reinforcing method, or even reinforcing-reducing method.

Position: Lateral position.

1. Guanyuan Acupoint

Location: In the lower abdomen, on the anterior midline, 3 cun (4-finger width) below the umbilicus.

Procedure: Heavy moxibustion with large moxa cones.

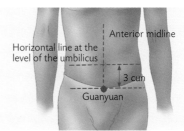

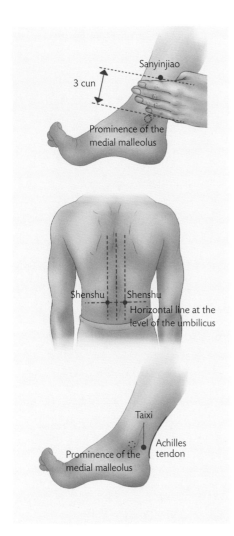

2. Sanyinjiao Acupoint

Location: On the medial aspect of the lower leg, 3 cun (4-finger width) above the prominence of the medial malleolus, posterior to the medial border of the tibia.

Procedure: Insert the needle perpendicularly into a depth of 1 to 1.5 cun, retaining it for 20 to 30 minutes (contraindicated during pregnancy).

3. Shenshu Acupoint

Location: In the lumbar region, at the same level as the inferior border of the spinous process of the 2nd lumbar vertebra, 1.5 cun lateral to the posterior midline.

Quick location: 2-finger width lateral to the intersection of the horizontal line at the level of the umbilicus and the spine.

Procedure: Insert the needle perpendicularly or obliquely into a depth of 0.5 to 1 cun, retaining it for 20 to 30 minutes.

4. Taixi Acupoint

Location: On the medial aspect of the foot, in the depression between the prominence of the lateral malleolus and the Achilles tendon.

Procedure: Insert the needle perpendicularly or obliquely into a depth of 0.5 to 1 cun, retaining it for 20 to 30 minutes.

Uterine Prolapse

Uterine prolapse refers to the descent of the uterus from its normal position along the vaginal canal, with the cervix extending below the level of the ischial spines, or even the complete protrusion of the uterus outside the vaginal orifice, or vaginal wall protrusion. The pathological focus of this condition is on the uterus, and acupuncture treatment aims to benefit *qi*, nourish the kidneys, and stabilize the uterus.

Acupuncture points: Baihui, Qihai, Dahe, Weidao, Zigong. Procedure: Conventional needle insertion. Position: Supine position.

1. Baihui Acupoint

Location: On the head, at the intersection of the line connecting both ear tips and the midline of the head.

Procedure: Insert the needle horizontally along the anterior-posterior direction, into a depth of 0.5 to 0.8 cun, retaining it for 20 to 30 minutes, applying acupuncture followed by moxibustion or applying them at the same time.

2. Qihai Acupoint

Location: On the anterior midline, 1.5 cun (about 2-finger width) below the umbilicus.

Procedure: Insert the needle obliquely into a depth of 1 to 1.5 cun, retaining it for 20 to 30 minutes.

3. Dahe Acupoint

Location: In the lower abdomen, 4 cun below the umbilicus, 0.5 cun lateral to the anterior midline, i.e., half-a-finger width lateral to Zhongji acupoint.

Procedure: Insert the needle perpendicularly into a depth of 1 to 1.5 cun, retaining it for 20 to 30 minutes.

4. Zigong Acupoint

Location: In the lower abdomen, 4 cun below the umbilicus, and 3 cun (4-finger width) lateral to the anterior midline.

Procedure: Insert the needle perpendicularly into a depth of 0.8 to 1.2 cun, retaining it for 20 to 30 minutes.

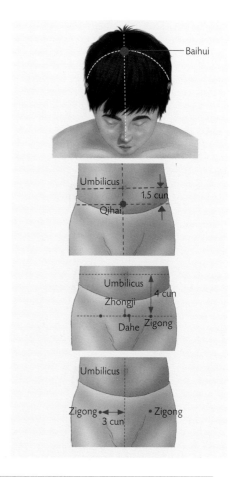

Physician's advice: ① Mild cases of uterine prolapse show significant acupuncture efficacy, while moderate to severe cases should combine acupuncture and medication for comprehensive treatment. ② During the treatment, instruct patients to perform levator ani muscle exercises. Before performing the exercises, ensure that the bowels are emptied. Contract the muscles around the anus as if holding back a bowel movement, holding for 5 seconds, then slowly relax the anal sphincter muscles. Rest for 10 seconds before repeating the sequence. Aim for around 40 to 50 repetitions daily, taking approximately 5 to 10 minutes each time. ③ Patients should rest adequately and avoid prolonged squatting or engaging in strenuous physical labor. ④ Sexual activity is prohibited during the treatment period.

Insufficient Lactation

This refers to the condition where lactating mothers produce little or no breast milk. The pathological focus of this condition is in the breasts. Acupuncture treatment focuses on regulating *qi* and blood, promoting the smooth flow of milk ducts.

Main acupuncture points include Danzhong , Rugen, and Shaoze. Specific acupuncture points for different patterns are as follows:

Patterns	Diagnostic Features	Acupuncture Points
Qi and blood deficiency	Dizziness, palpitations, pale complexion, lack of luster in lips and nails, pale tongue with thin coating	Main acupoints + Pishu, Zusanli
Liver depression and phlegm binding	Emotional repression, chest tightness, excessive phlegm	Main acupoints + Taichong, Fenglong

Procedure: Conventional needle insertion.

Position: Supine position.

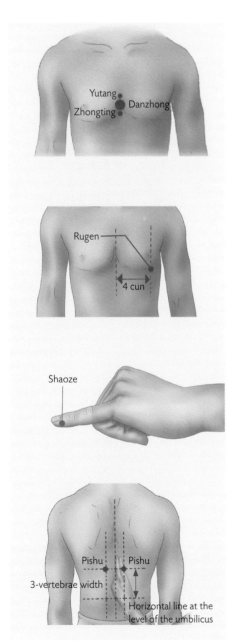

Main Acupoints

1. Danzhong Acupoint

Location: At the midpoint between the nipples, horizontally at the 4th intercostal space.

Procedure: Employ the skin-pinching up needle inserting method, horizontally insert the needle into the chests at both sides with a depth of 0.3 to 0.5 cun, retaining it for 20 to 30 minutes.

2. Rugen Acupoint

Location: In the chest, precisely below the nipple, at the base of the breast, in the 5th intercostal space, 4 cun (about 5-finger width) lateral to the anterior midline.

Procedure: Horizontally insert the needle into the base of the breast with a depth of 0.5 to 0.8 cun to make a slight swelling sensation, retaining it for 20 to 30 minutes.

3. Shaoze Acupoint

Location: On the medial end of the little finger, 0.1 cun from the corner of the nail.

Procedure: Insert the needle shallowly into a depth of 0.1 cun.

Qi and Blood Deficiency: Main Acupoints + Pishu, Zusanli

1. Pishu Acupoint

Location: On the back, below the spinous process of the 11th thoracic vertebra, 1.5 cun lateral to the posterior midline.

Quick location: 3 vertebrae above the intersection of the horizontal line at the level of the umbilicus and the spine, 2-finger width lateral to the lower edge.

Procedure: Insert the needle perpendicularly or obliquely into a depth of 0.5 to 1 cun, retaining it for 20 to 30 minutes.

2. Zusanli Acupoint

Location: On the front lateral aspect of the lower leg, 3 cun (about 4-finger width) below the Dubi acupoint, 1-finger width lateral to the anterior crest of the tibia.

Quick location: Stand and bend over; use the tiger's mouth of hand on the same side to encircle the upper lateral border of the patella, with the remaining 4 fingers pointing downward, and the tip of the middle finger is this acupoint.

Procedure: Insert the needle perpendicularly or obliquely into a depth of 0.5 to 1 cun, retaining it for 20 to 30 minutes.

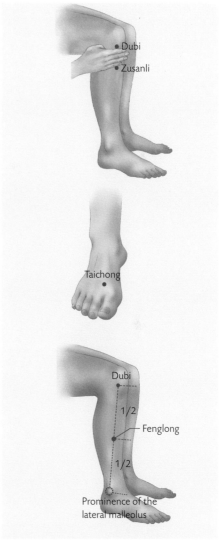

Liver Depression and Phlegm Binding: Main Acupoints + Taichong, Fenglong

1. Taichong Acupoint

Location: On the dorsum of the foot, at the depression in front of the junction between the 1st and 2nd metatarsal bones.

Quick location: On the dorsum of the foot, push upward along the crease between the 1st and 2nd toes. The depression felt is the Taichong acupoint.

Procedure: Insert the needle perpendicularly into a depth of 0.5 to 0.8 cun, retaining it for 20 to 30 minutes.

2. Fenglong Acupoint

Location: On the front lateral aspect of the lower leg, 8 cun above the lateral malleolus, 2-finger width from the anterior edge of the tibia.

Quick location: Bend the knee, draw a line between Dubi acupoint and the lateral malleolus, and find the midpoint of the line.

Procedure: Insert the needle perpendicularly or obliquely into a depth of 0.5 to 1 cun, retaining it for 20 to 30 minutes.

 Physician's advice: ① During the treatment period, advise patients to regulate their emotions, enhance nutrition, avoid excessive fatigue, and ensure sufficient sleep. ② For cases of milk stasis or breast pain, instruct patients to avoid squeezing the breasts to prevent the occurrence of acute mastitis.

CHAPTER SEVEN
Acupuncture Treatment for Ophthalmological, Otorhinolaryngological, and Stomatological Conditions

This chapter covers common ophthalmology conditions such as myopia, sore throat, toothache, etc. Note that acupuncture should be performed by professionals. Please exercise caution, and ensure that the intensity of acupuncture is within the patient's comfort level.

Myopia

Myopia is an ocular condition, clinically identified by clear vision of nearby objects contrasted with blurry vision of distant objects and a decline in visual acuity. The pathological focus of this condition is in the eyes, attributed to stagnation of ocular meridians and subsequent deprivation of ocular nourishment. Acupuncture therapy aims to clear and activate collaterals, and promote visual clarity.

Acupuncture points: Jingming, Chengqi, Sibai, Taiyang, Fengchi, Guangming.

Procedure: Conventional needle insertion.

Position: Supine position.

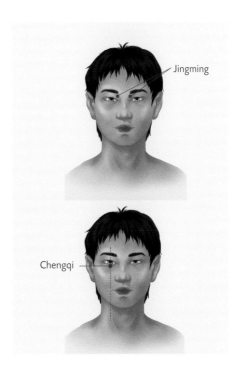

1. Jingming Acupoint

Location: On the face, in the depression slightly above the medial angle of the eye.

Procedure: Instruct the patient to close eyes. Use the left hand to stabilize the eyeball outward, and use the right hand to gently insert the needle perpendicularly along the edge of the orbit into a depth of 0.5 to 1 cun. Do not lift-thrust or twirl the needle. Retain the needle for 20 to 30 minutes. After withdrawing the needle, press the needle hole for a moment.

2. Chengqi Acupoint

Location: On the face, directly below the pupil while looking straight ahead, between the eyeball and the lower margin of the orbit.

Procedure: Instruct the patient to close

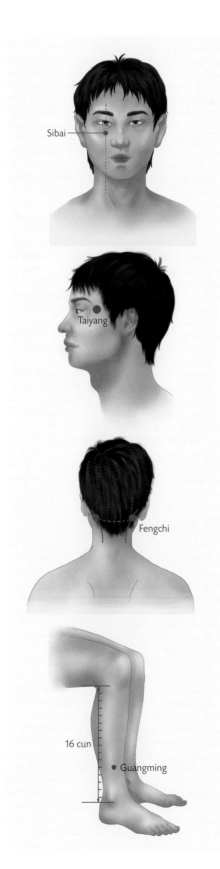

Sibai

Taiyang

Fengchi

16 cun

Guangming

eyes. Use the left hand to stabilize the eyeball outward, and use the right hand to gently insert the needle perpendicularly along the edge of the orbit into a depth of 0.5 to 1 cun. Do not lift-thrust or twirl the needle. Retain the needle for 20 to 30 minutes. After withdrawing the needle, press the needle hole for a moment.

3. Sibai Acupoint

Location: On the face, directly below the pupil while looking straight ahead, in the depression of the foramina infraorbitale.

Procedure: Insert the needle perpendicularly into a depth of 0.3 to 0.5 cun, retaining it for 20 to 30 minutes.

4. Taiyang Acupoint

Location: In the temporal region of the head, between the tip of the eyebrow and the outer canthus, in the depression approximately 1-finger width backwards.

Procedure: Insert the needle perpendicularly into a depth of 0.3 to 0.5 cun, retaining it for 20 to 30 minutes.

5. Fengchi Acupoint

Location: In the posterior neck region, below the occipital bone, in the depression between the upper end of the sternocleidomastoid muscle and the trapezius muscle.

Quick location: Sit upright, and the acupoint is situated in the depression on the lateral edge of the two major tendons below the occipital bone, level with the earlobe.

Procedure: Insert the needle obliquely towards the tip of the nose with the tip of the needle slightly downward, into a depth of 0.5 to 0.8 cun, or insert the needle horizontally towards the Fengfu acupoint (see page 133), retaining it for 20 to 30 minutes.

6. Guangming Acupoint

Location: On the lateral aspect of the lower leg, 5 cun above the prominence of the lateral malleolus, along the anterior edge of the fibula.

Procedure: Insert the needle obliquely upward into a depth of 1 to 1.5 cun, guiding the needling sensation upwards, and retaining the needle for 20 to 30 minutes.

Physician's advice: ① Acupuncture shows remarkable efficacy in treating pseudomyopia, with higher cure rates observed in younger patients.
② Maintain good eye hygiene in daily routines. ③ Take regular measures to safeguard vision and prevent prolonged eye strain.

Paralytic Strabismus

Strabismus refers to the condition where one or both eyes deviate inwards or outwards when focusing on a target, resulting in limited eye movement and double vision. It is more prevalent in children. The pathological focus of this condition is in the eyes, the acupuncture treatment focuses on suppressing hyperactive liver for calming endogenous wind, promoting blood circulation and activating collaterals. The treatment demonstrates remarkable efficacy, particularly in patients with a short disease duration.

The main acupuncture points include Fengchi, Sibai, Cuanzhu, Tongziliao, and Yanglingquan. Specific acupuncture points for different patterns are as follows:

Patterns	Diagnostic Features	Acupuncture Points
Invasion of wind pathogen	Sudden onset, accompanied by headache or dizziness, droopy upper eyelid, chills and fever	Main acupoints + Fengfu
Liver wind stirring up internally	Dizziness, tinnitus, flushed face, restlessness, limb numbness and tremors	Main acupoints + Ganshu
Static blood obstruction and stagnation	Mostly with history of traumas, blood stasis in the whites of the eyes, headache, eye swelling, nausea, and vomiting	Main acupoints + Geshu

Procedure: Conventional needle insertion.
Position: Sitting position.

Main Acupoints

1. Fengchi Acupoint
Location: In the posterior neck region, below the occipital bone, in the depression between the upper end of the sternocleidomastoid muscle and the trapezius muscle.

Quick location: Sit upright, and the acupoint is situated in the depression on the lateral edge of the two major tendons below the occipital bone, level with the earlobe.

Procedure: Insert the needle obliquely

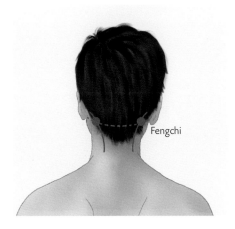

Fengchi

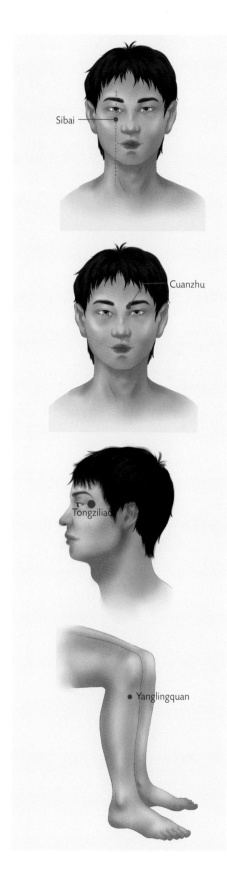

towards the tip of the nose, into a depth of
0.5 to 0.8 cun with the tip of the needle slightly
downward, or insert the needle horizontally
towards the Fengfu acupoint (see page 133),
retaining it for 20 to 30 minutes.

2. Sibai Acupoint

Location: On the face, directly below
the pupil while looking straight ahead, in the
depression of the foramina infraorbitale.

Procedure: Insert the needle
perpendicularly into a depth of 0.3 to 0.5 cun,
retaining it for 20 to 30 minutes.

3. Cuanzhu Acupoint

Location: In the depression at the inner tip
of the eyebrows, at the supraorbital notch.

Procedure: Insert the needle horizontally or
obliquely towards the middle of the eyebrow or
the inner edge of the orbit, into a depth of 0.5 to
0.8 cun, retaining it for 20 to 30 minutes.

4. Tongziliao Acupoint

Location: On the face, next to the tail of the
eye, at the outer edge of the orbit.

Procedure: Insert the needle horizontally
towards the Taiyang acupoint (see page 130) into
a depth of 0.5 to 1 cun, retaining it for 20 to 30
minutes.

5. Yanglingquan Acupoint

Location: On the lateral aspect of the
lower leg, in the depression below the anterior
capitulum fibulae.

Procedure: Insert the needle
perpendicularly or obliquely into a depth of
0.5 to 1 cun, retaining it for 20 to 30 minutes.

**Invasion of Wind Pathogen: Main Acupoints
+ Fengfu**

Fengfu Acupoint

Location: On the nape, 1 cun (1-finger width)
above the posterior hairline, directly below the
external occipital protuberance, in the depression
between the two trapeziuses.

Procedure: Slowly insert the needle in a

downward direction towards the lower mandible into a depth of 0.5 to 1 cun, avoiding upward deep insertion and retaining the needle for 20 to 30 minutes.

Liver Wind Stirring up Internally: Main Acupoints + Ganshu

Ganshu Acupoint

Location: On the back, below the spinous process of the 9th thoracic vertebra, 1.5 cun lateral to the posterior midline.

Quick location: 2 vertebrae below the intersection of the horizontal line drawn from the inferior angle of the scapula and the spine (the spinous process of the 7th thoracic vertebra), 2-finger width lateral to the lower edge.

Procedure: Insert the needle obliquely into a depth of 0.5 to 0.8 cun, retaining it for 20 to 30 minutes.

Static Blood Obstruction and Stagnation: Main Acupoints + Geshu

Geshu Acupoint

Location: On the back, below the spinous process of the 7th thoracic vertebra, 1.5 cun lateral to the posterior midline.

Quick location: The intersection of the horizontal line drawn from the inferior angle of the scapula and the spine (the spinous process of the 7th thoracic vertebra), 2-finger width lateral to the lower edge.

Procedure: Insert the needle perpendicularly or obliquely into a depth of 0.5 to 1 cun, retaining it for 20 to 30 minutes.

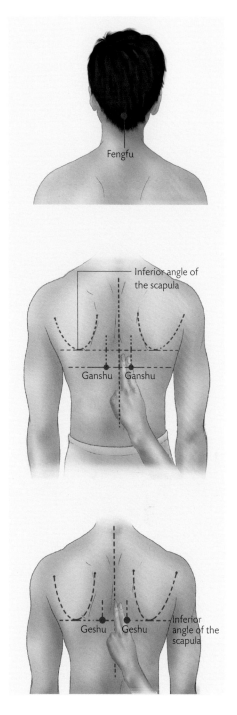

Blepharoptosis

Blepharoptosis is a condition characterized by the weakened or inability of the upper eyelid to lift properly, resulting in a narrowed palpebral fissure that may partially or completely cover the pupil, thus affecting vision. The pathological focus of this condition is in the muscles of the eyelids. Acupuncture treatment focuses on invigorating spleen

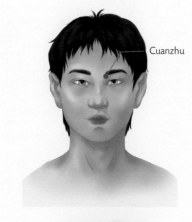

Cuanzhu

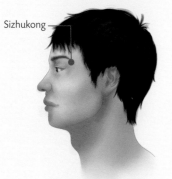

Sizhukong

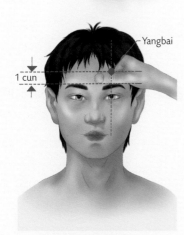

Yangbai

1 cun

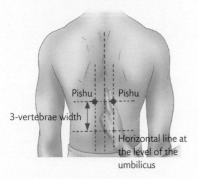

Pishu | Pishu

3-vertebrae width

Horizontal line at
the level of the
umbilicus

and enhancing *qi* circulation, nourishing the blood and strengthening the muscles. In cases of congenital severe blepharoptosis, surgical intervention may be considered.

Acupuncture points: Cuanzhu, Sizhukong, Yangbai, Pishu, Shenshu, Sanyinjiao

Procedure: Conventional needle insertion.

Position: Lateral position.

1. Cuanzhu Acupoint

Location: In the depression at the inner tip of the eyebrows, at the supraorbital notch.

Procedure: Insert the needle horizontally or obliquely towards the middle of the eyebrow or the inner edge of the orbit, into a depth of 0.5 to 0.8 cun, retaining it for 20 to 30 minutes.

2. Sizhukong Acupoint

Location: In the depression at the tip of the eyebrow.

Procedure: Insert the needle horizontally into a depth of 0.3 to 0.5 cun, retaining it for 20 to 30 minutes.

3. Yangbai Acupoint

Location: On the forehead, directly above the pupil, 1 cun (1-finger width) above the eyebrow.

Procedure: Utilize the skin-pinching up needle inserting method, and insert the needle horizontally towards the pupil direction into a depth of 0.5 to 0.8 cun, retaining it for 20 to 30 minutes.

4. Pishu Acupoint

Location: On the back, below the spinous process of the 11th thoracic vertebra, 1.5 cun lateral to the posterior midline.

Quick location: 3 vertebrae above the intersection of the horizontal line at the level of the umbilicus and the spine, 2-finger width lateral to the lower edge.

Procedure: Insert the needle perpendicularly or obliquely into a depth of 0.5 to 1 cun, retaining it for 20 to 30 minutes.

5. Shenshu Acupoint

Location: In the lumbar region, below the spinous process of the 2nd lumbar vertebra, 1.5 cun lateral to the posterior midline.

Quick location: 2-finger width lateral to the intersection of the horizontal line at the level of the umbilicus and the spine.

Procedure: Insert the needle perpendicularly or obliquely into a depth of 0.5 to 1 cun, retaining it for 20 to 30 minutes.

6. Sanyinjiao Acupoint

Location: On the medial aspect of the lower leg, 3 cun (4-finger width) above the prominence of the medial malleolus, posterior to the medial border of the tibia.

Procedure: Utilize the even reinforcing-reducing method, lifting-thrusting reinforcing method or twirling reinforcing method, and insert the needle perpendicularly or obliquely into a depth of 0.5 to 1 cun; retain the needle for 20 to 30 minutes.

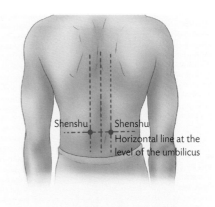

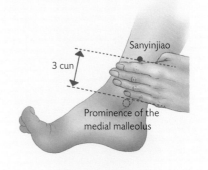

Sore Throat

Sore throat, often associated with pharyngitis or tonsillitis, manifests as redness, swelling, heat, pain, and discomfort while swallowing in the throat region. The pathological focus of this condition is in the throat. Specific acupuncture points for different patterns are as follows:

Patterns	Diagnostic Features	Acupuncture Points
Scorching sensation due to fire-heat	Redness, swelling, heat, and pain in the throat, discomfort while swallowing, fever, constipation, yellow urine	Shaoshang, Shangyang, Tianrong, Guanchong, Neiting
Hyperactivity of fire due to *yin* deficiency	Dry and slightly painful throat, exacerbated in the afternoon or evening, heat sensations in the palms and soles, red tongue with little coating	Taixi, Zhaohai, Lieque, Yuji

Procedure: For scorching sensation due to fire-heat, utilize lifting-thrusting reducing method or twirling reducing method; for hyperactivity of fire due to *yin* deficiency, employ lifting-thrusting reinforcing method, twirling reinforcing method, or even reinforcing-reducing method. During the needling process at the Lieque and Zhaohai points, the patient can be guided to swallow as instructed by the physician.

Position: Supine position.

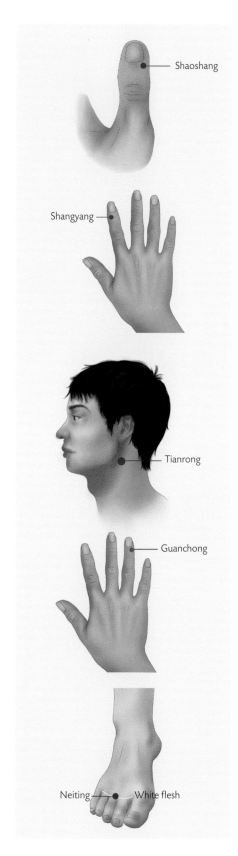

Shaoshang

Shangyang

Tianrong

Guanchong

Neiting — White flesh

Scorching Sensation Due to Fire-Heat

1. Shaoshang Acupoint

Location: On the lateral aspect of the distal phalanx of the thumb, 0.1 cun from the corner of the nail.

Procedure: Insert the needle shallowly into a depth of 0.1 cun, retaining it for 20 to 30 minutes.

2. Shangyang Acupoint

Positioning: On the radial side of the distal phalanx of the index finger, 0.1 cun from the corner of the nail.

Procedure: Insert the needle shallowly into a depth of 0.1 cun, retaining it for 20 to 30 minutes.

3. Tianrong Acupoint

Location: On the lateral aspect of the neck, posterior to the angle of mandible, in the depression of the anterior edge of the sternocleidomastoid muscle.

Procedure: Insert the needle obliquely into a depth of 0.5 to 0.8 cun, ensuring avoidance of blood vessels, and retain the needle for 20 to 30 minutes.

4. Guanchong Acupoint

Position: On the ulnar side of the distal phalanx of the ring finger, 0.1 cun from the corner of the nail.

Procedure: Insert the needle shallowly into a depth of 0.1 cun, retaining it for 20 to 30 minutes.

5. Neiting Acupoint

Location: On the dorsum of the foot, between the 2nd and 3rd toes, at the junction of the red and white flesh posterior to the toe web.

Procedure: Insert the needle perpendicularly or obliquely into a depth of 0.5 to 1 cun, retaining it for 20 to 30 minutes.

Hyperactivity of Fire Due to *Yin* Deficiency

1. Taixi Acupoint

Location: On the medial aspect of the foot, in the depression between the prominence of the lateral malleolus and the Achilles tendon.

Procedure: Insert the needle perpendicularly or obliquely into a depth of 0.5 to 1 cun, retaining it for 20 to 30 minutes.

2. Zhaohai Acupoint

Location: On the medial aspect of the foot, 1 cun below the prominence of the medial malleolus in the depression.

Procedure: Insert the needle perpendicularly or obliquely into a depth of 0.5 to 1 cun, retaining it for 20 to 30 minutes.

3. Lieque Acupoint

Location: Cross the hands naturally with the tiger's mouth of hand, and press one index finger on the styloid process of the radius (the high prominence on the thumb side behind the wrist). The acupuncture point is located under the fingertip of the index finger.

Procedure: Insert the needle perpendicularly or obliquely into a depth of 0.5 to 1 cun, retaining it for 20 to 30 minutes.

4. Yuji Acupoint

Location: Posterior to the 1st metacarpophalangeal joint, at the junction of the red and white flesh on the radial side of the midpoint of the 1st metacarpal bone.

Procedure: Insert the needle perpendicularly or obliquely into a depth of 0.5 to 1 cun, retaining it for 20 to 30 minutes.

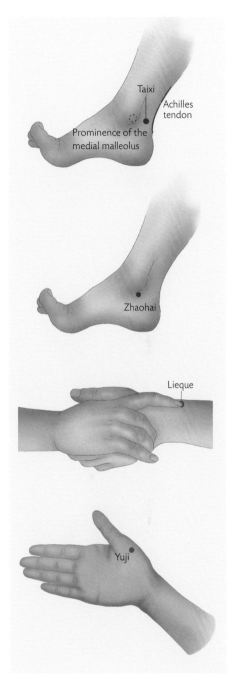

Physician's advice: ① Acupuncture is more effective for sore throat with scorching sensation due to fire-heat. ② Patients should avoid consuming spicy and irritating foods, quit smoking and drinking, and steer clear of harmful gases. ③ If there is purulence around the tonsils or if acute laryngitis presents with swelling and difficulty breathing, seeking specialized treatment at the hospital is advised.

Toothache

Toothache, the most prevalent oral condition, refers to pain arising from various causes within the teeth. The pathological focus of this condition is in the throat, and acupuncture treatment focuses on dispelling wind-evil and purging fire, activating collaterals and alleviating discomfort.

The main acupuncture points include Jiache, Xiaguan, Hegu, and Neiting. Specific acupuncture points for different patterns are as follows:

Patterns	Diagnostic Features	Acupuncture Points
Toothache due to wind-fire	Sudden onset, severe toothache, red and swollen gums, preference for cold and aversion to heat, accompanied by fever	Main acupoints + Yifeng
Toothache due to stomach fire	Severe toothache, red and swollen gums, even bleeding, accompanied by bad breath, constipation, and yellow urine	Main acupoints + Lidui
Toothache due to deficiency-fire	Dull pain, exacerbating in the afternoon or at night, persisting without relief over time with gum recession and teeth loosening	Main acupoints + Taixi

Procedure: Utilize lifting-thrusting reducing method or twirling reducing method.
Position: Supine position.

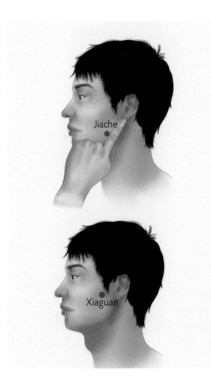

Main Acupoints

1. Jiache Acupoint

Location: On the face, in the depression when the masseter muscle bulges during chewing.

Quick location: On the face, 1-finger width (middle finger) above the anterior superior angle of the mandible.

Procedure: Insert the needle perpendicularly into a depth of 0.3 to 0.5 cun, or insert the needle horizontally into a depth of 1 to 1.5 cun towards the direction of Dicang acupoint (see page 61), retaining it for 20 to 30 minutes.

2. Xiaguan Acupoint

Location: In front of the ear, in the depression formed by the lower edge of the zygomatic arch and the mandibular notch.

Quick location: Sit or lie on the side, close

the mouth, and identify the point about 1-finger width in front of the tragus, in the depression below the zygomatic arch.

Procedure: Insert the needle perpendicularly into a depth of 0.5 to 1 cun, ensuring the mouth remains closed during needling, and retain the needle for 20 to 30 minutes.

3. Hegu Acupoint

Location: On the dorsum of the hand, between the 1st and 2nd metacarpal bones, at the midpoint of the radial side on the 2nd metacarpal bone.

Quick location: Take the crease of the thumb interphalangeal joint of one hand and place it on the edge of the web between the thumb and forefinger of the other hand, where the tip of the thumb lands is Hegu acupoint.

Procedure: Insert the needle perpendicularly or obliquely into a depth of 0.5 to 1 cun, retaining it for 20 to 30 minutes.

4. Neiting Acupoint

Location: On the dorsum of the foot, between the 2nd and 3rd toes, at the junction of the red and white flesh posterior to the toe web.

Procedure: Insert the needle perpendicularly or obliquely into a depth of 0.5 to 1 cun, retaining it for 20 to 30 minutes. Alternatively, peck needling method can also be applied, which is short-term, high-frequency needling without needle retention to induce bleeding.

Toothache Due to Wind-Fire: Main Acupoints + Yifeng

Yifeng Acupoint

Location: Posterior to the earlobe, in the depression behind between the mastoid process and the angle of mandible.

Quick location: Pressing behind the earlobe, locate the depression within its covered area, which corresponds to this acupoint.

Procedure: Insert the needle perpendicularly into a depth of 0.5 to 1 cun, retaining it for 20 to 30 minutes.

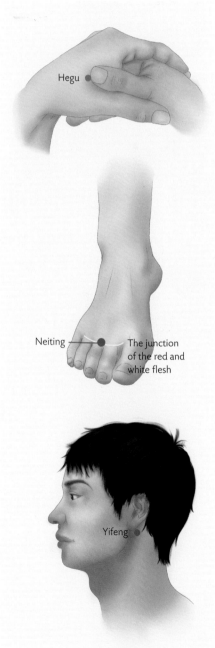

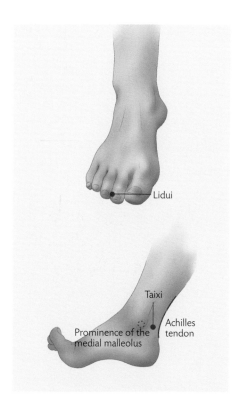

Toothache Due to Stomach Fire: Main Acupoints + Lidui

Lidui Acupoint

Location: On the lateral aspect of the distal phalanx of the 2nd toe, 0.1 cun from the corner of the nail.

Procedure: Insert the needle shallowly into a depth of 0.1 cun, retaining it for 20 to 30 minutes.

Toothache Due to Deficiency-Fire: Main Acupoint + Taixi

Taixi Acupoint

Location: On the medial aspect of the foot, in the depression between the prominence of the lateral malleolus and the Achilles tendon.

Procedure: Insert the needle perpendicularly or obliquely into a depth of 0.5 to 1 cun, retaining it for 20 to 30 minutes.

Physician's advice: ① Maintain good oral hygiene and avoid extreme temperatures and acidic or sweet foods. ② Be mindful of distinguishing symptoms from trigeminal neuralgia. ③ For patients who have undergone 3 to 5 treatment courses with about 50 acupuncture sessions and still have no improvement, it is important to investigate the cause of the condition.